Contents

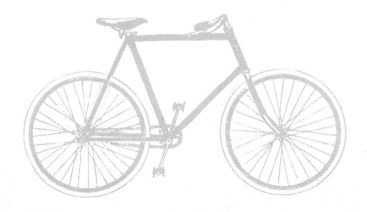

For Ariel,

who gave us the idea for this book

on a hot summer Sunday

FIRESIDE
Rockefeller Center
1230 Avenue of the Americas
New York, NY 10020

DESIGNED BY BARBARA MARKS
MAPS BY DANIEL CHIU

Manufactured in the United States of America

10 9 8 7 6 5 4 3 2

Library of Congress Cataloging-in-Publication Data
Williams, Wendy
    The best bike paths of New England / Wendy Williams.
        p.   cm.
    "A Fireside book."
    1. Bicycle touring—New England—Guidebooks.   2. Bicycle trails—
New England—Guidebooks.   3. New England—Guidebooks.   I. Title.
GV1045.5.N36W45   1995
796.6'4'0974—dc20   95-50018
                                                              CIP

ISBN 0-684-81399-8

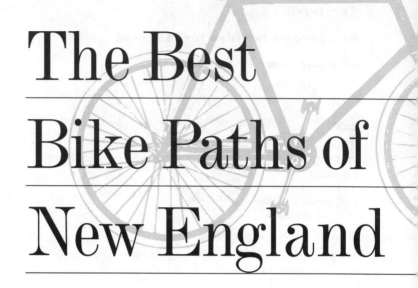

The Best
Bike Paths of
New England

Wendy Williams

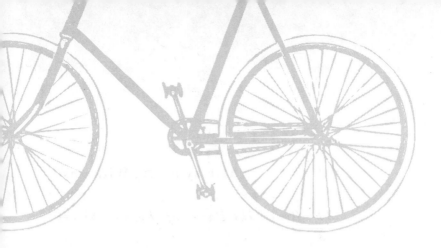

Safe, Scenic, and

Traffic-Free Bicycling

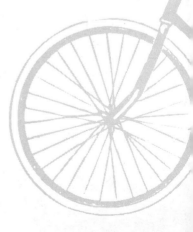

A Fireside Book

Published by Simon & Schuster

New York London Toronto Sydney Tokyo Singapore

Also by Wendy Williams:

The Best Bike Paths of the Southwest

Introduction

O n Cape Cod, you can crest a sand dune and look for whales in the Atlantic Ocean. Far from the maddening crowd and the traffic-filled roads, you can coast down the bike path to rest in the shade of a pine tree or sit by the shore and listen to the waves.

In New Hampshire, while others contend with cars and crowds, your family can see Franconia Notch State Park by riding the 10-mile paved path. You'll cross the river on bikes-only bridges, stop to rest on the banks of crystal-clear lakes, cool off by wading in ice-cold streams.

In Maine, at Acadia National Park, you can pedal along miles of carriage roads. Closed to automobiles, these historic roads include lakeside rambles easy enough for 5-year-olds or mountainside climbs for those in top physical shape.

You can see Boston or Burlington from a bike path, or Hartford or Narragansett Bay. All across America, miles of these exquisite paved paths are being built each month. This burgeoning network is creating a new form of biking, bringing "accessible adventure" to families, enabling parents with young children or older adults to plan safe and scenic bike rides through some of America's most beautiful settings.

But where are they? America's paved-path network is a grass-roots system, built bit by bit, as various groups and people have become involved. Sponsoring organizations have included the federal Department of Transportation, the National Park Service, state transportation departments and state parks, small municipalities, community activist groups, and even, in a few cases, private organizations funded by individual donations.

Because of this diversity, a comprehensive listing and description of America's paved paths simply hasn't existed. In this book, we've provided the information you'll need to find these hidden treasures. Whether you're a parent planning an outing with young children, an avid cyclist who thinks a 50-mile ride is a short day's work, or an older adult (like me) back in the saddle after a long hiatus—you'll be able to read this book and pick out the rides best suited to you and your cycling companions.

How to Use This Book:

At the beginning of each listing, we've included a few facts to let you know quickly the basic parameters of that particular path: a descriptive sentence that usually includes the one-way length of the path, the level of difficulty, the type of scenery you'll be riding through, and the condition of the path.

We realize that "level of difficulty" is a matter of personal opinion. The 3 descriptions we've used—"Easy," "Average," "Challenging"—are based on the experiences of us: a group of friends, mostly in their mid-40s, who ride once or twice a week on a casual basis. If you are a distance cyclist, you may find some of our "challenging" rides to be rather easy; if you are a parent with a 5-year-old, you may find our "average" rides too difficult. Scale up or down, according to your abilities and interests.

At the end of each entry, we've listed a contact address and telephone number. Many paths in this book are in transition right now, being lengthened or rebuilt or otherwise improved. For the most up-to-date information, we suggest you contact the listed agency. Sometimes these agencies can also help you with other questions, including where to stay or what other activities might be available.

Rules of the Road and Other Necessities:

Most states now have laws requiring children to wear helmets when cycling. We suggest that helmets are appropriate for everyone.

Also good to bring: plenty of water, a quick-energy snack, a tire-patch kit, a first-aid kit, and a bike lock.

In general, bike and recreation paths are like automobile roads. The rules are pretty much the same. Usually everyone is asked to keep to the right; to signal when passing; to maintain reasonable speed limits; and to respect the rights of others. If you are riding with friends, don't ride abreast, blocking the way for others. If you stop to rest, pull off the path onto the shoulder. Some of the newer paths even have scenic rest areas, attractive places with benches or picnic tables where you can talk, eat, or make repairs without impeding traffic.

Recreation paths are not appropriate places for high-speed cycling. They are for recreation and welcome anyone, from children on tricycles to seniors out for a stroll. Acceptable speeds range from about 5 miles per hour to about 20 miles per hour.

A Word to In-Line Skaters:

In-line skaters and cyclists coexist comfortably on today's wide recreation paths; most paths in this book welcome in-line skaters and walkers as well as cyclists. In the few places where we have seen skating expressly forbidden (on the Cape Cod National Seashore paths and the Franconia Notch State Park path, for example) we have mentioned the restriction. However, this can change. If you want to skate on a particular path, we suggest you check ahead to be sure.

Keep in mind that recreation paths are *not* appropriate places to teach young children how to skate or cycle; we've seen serious accidents result when tottering children fell in front of oncoming cyclists.

In California, where we saw some astonishingly facile skaters, cyclists and skaters mixed happily, making room for each other's styles with gracious acceptance. All it takes is mutual tolerance. The cyclists respected the skaters' need for extra sideways maneuverability, while the skaters moved over quickly when faster cyclists called out politely from behind.

The Best
Bike Paths of
New England

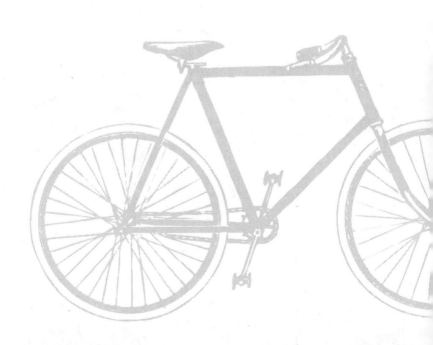

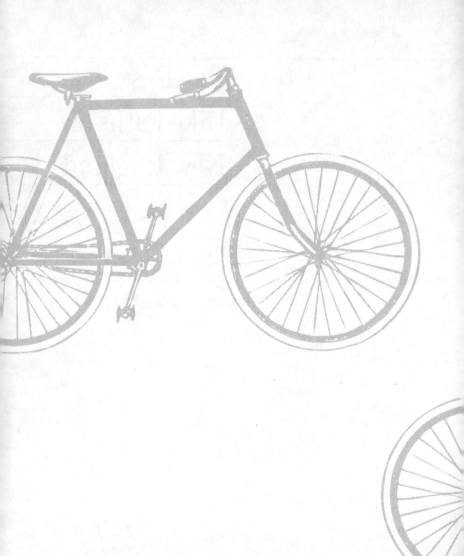

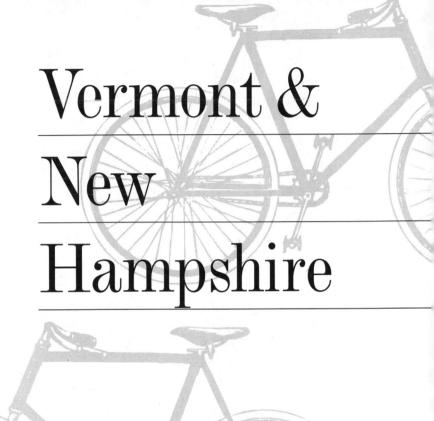

Vermont &
New
Hampshire

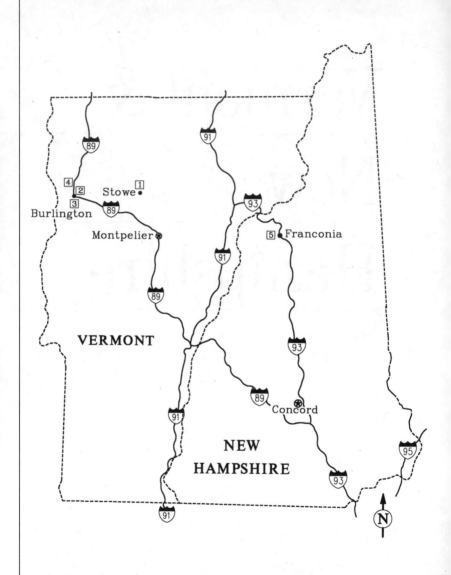

Vermont &
New Hampshire

1. The Stowe Recreation Path

General Description:

A 5.3-mile path, enhancing the soft, natural beauty of the Green Mountains, winner of many design awards; called the "119th Point of Light" by the Bush administration.

Level of Difficulty: Average.

Type of Scenery: The village of Stowe, where the Trapp family lives; dairy farms and flower-filled fields; Mount Mansfield, the state's tallest mountain; the meandering West Branch River; 11 softly arched wooden bridges.

Condition of Pavement: Excellent.

General Background:

This path sets the standard for natural beauty and thoughtful elegance. When it comes to laying out paths that reflect the area's natural grace, Stowe is tops.

The ride follows the course of the twisting West Branch River, a stream flowing out of the Green Mountains. It would have been simpler and cheaper to lay the pavement in a straight line along one bank of the river, but designers didn't do that.

Instead, imitating the mountain stream, the path snakes through forestland and pasturage, crossing and recrossing the real stream on softly arched wooden bridges, so that the recreation path and the West Branch River entwine in intimate embrace.

Adorning the path are examples of the Vermont ethic of simple country elegance. We saw a charming cupola in one small field. Wooden benches are plentiful. Well-designed stone walls mark off territory at several points. Delicately lettered signs along the trail, pointing out inns and restaurants, are often so tiny as to be barely visible. Even the "rules" in the path brochure—not called "rules" at all, but "user ethics"—are worded with great finesse: "4. Please suggest to your dogs that they use the woods."

Nothing on the trail mars the Green Mountain scenery or spoils the fun. The people of Stowe obviously cherish their path: even the herd of black-and-white dairy cows standing in their Sunday-morning mountain pasturage seemed to have been groomed and placed just so, to perfect the scene.

From the beginning, this path has enjoyed exceptional local support. A local agency first began discussing the benefits of a recreation path in 1964, but nothing was done until 1977, when a private citizen paid the state Highway Department to design a bike path. That completed design lay dormant until the town hired a part-time recreation activist, Anne Lusk, in 1981.

Lusk proved to be a dynamo. First garnering community and citizen support, she convinced 32 private landowners to grant deeds of easement over their properties. Some of these landowners were restaurateurs and innkeepers who stood to profit from a well-used recreation path, but others apparently helped just because the community values the area's natural beauty.

In keeping with this grass-roots support, the names of all the path's donors are listed in large books placed at points along the path. Hundreds of individuals and businesses are listed: those who made large contributions and those who contributed on the smaller scale of $2 per inch.

The Bike Path:

This is one of the few New England paths with a definite, if gradual, direction of incline. Beginning in Stowe, just behind the large white church at the center of town, the path climbs into the mountains, ending at a wooden bridge on Brook Road, just off Mountain Road. Because of the many small dips and hills along the path, the incline is not obvious, but it is there. Most people will be able to bike up the path, taking advantage of the frequent dips for a short downhill coast. On the return ride, you'll relax by coasting much of the way back down.

If you have the energy to bike up and back, we suggest you do. We promise: you won't be bored. Begin in the large recreation-path parking area behind the Stowe Community Church. At about a quarter-mile, when the path curves through some pine trees, look back across the well-maintained lawns toward the church and enjoy the classic New England scenery. For the next mile or so, you'll pedal easily along the stream and enjoy the plantings maintained by the local garden club. The path here has a minimal incline.

After crossing Weeks Hill Road, the path begins

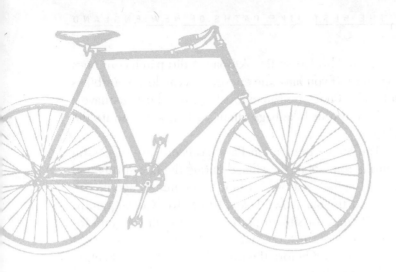

climbing a bit more steeply, although not forbiddingly. Biking along this segment, you'll be nearer the commercial area of town. Don't despair: This is only temporary. When you leave this short stretch of stores and restaurants, the ride is better than ever. At about midpoint, you'll cross the highway, Mountain Road, or Route 108.

Riding out of town, the path was pleasingly pretty; now it takes on an esthetic grace, bending and twisting with its own personal rhythm through the countryside. Far from the highway and stores, you'll see open fields filled with wildflowers in the summertime; in the fall, you'll ride through a cacophony of color, as the leaves fall from the maple and oak and birch trees.

In the distance stands Mount Mansfield, with its lacing of downhill ski trails. As you continue, you'll cross more bridges and pass a riding stable. The paved road ends at the covered bridge on Brook Road. A dirt patch continues from here. If you have the energy, you can lock your bikes and walk. If not, you can enjoy the covered bridge, have a snack from your bike bags, then coast back down into the village.

The Stowe Recreation Path has been very successful in luring tourists to the village during the late spring and late fall "quiet seasons," when the summer people are gone and the ski crowd has yet to arrive. Consequently, plans abound for similar paths in nearby villages, and for an extension of the Stowe path itself. Some of these might come to fruition before the turn of the century, but action doesn't seem imminent.

Very near this recreation path are a school and camp for in-line skating. Skaters make full use of this recreation path.

Food Facilities Nearby: Restaurants, sandwich shops, and delis, all along the path. Whatever you need won't be far away.

Restrooms: In the village, there are public restrooms at The Stowe Area Association, Main Street across from Shaw's General Store; Town Hall, Main Street, Stowe Village. Several port-o-potties at the upper end of the path.

Special Precautions: Remember the slight uphill incline. If you're not used to 10-mile cycling trips, start at the top, at the covered bridge on Brook Road, and enjoy the trip down.

Best Parking Lot: The ample parking lots along the path are not always easy to find, because the signs are intentionally unobtrusive. You can park in the large lot directly behind the white church on Main Street, in the center of Stowe; at the Luce Hill Road path parking lot, off Mountain Road near Cottage Club Road; at the Mountain Road parking lot, toward the path's end.

Directions: Take Route 100 into the village of Stowe. If you're coming from Interstate 89, you'll enter the village and see Mountain Road or Route 108 branching to the left. To get to the church parking lot, continue instead a very short distance along Route 100 until you see the white steeple of the church. Turn left into the parking lot.

To get to the other parking lots, turn left up Mountain Road. In about a mile, begin looking for Luce Hill Road on the left. The Mountain Road parking lot is also on the left, farther up the road. Brook Road is also a left turn off Mountain Road.

For More Information: The Stowe Area Association, P.O. Box 1320, Main Street, Stowe, Vermont 05672. Tel.: (802) 253-6617; (800) 24-STOWE.

2. The Burlington Bikeway

General Description:

A 7.1-mile path following the rugged shore of Lake Champlain.

Level of Difficulty: Easy.

Type of Scenery: The shore of Lake Champlain, with the mountains of New York State in the distance; distant islands often shadowed by fog and clouds; 7 waterfront parks with public swimming areas; some urban and suburban areas; the Winooski River.

Condition of Pavement: Excellent.

General Background:

Burlington began life as a small farming village, quiet and pristine, nestled onto a small section of shoreline on Lake Champlain, that huge body of water that marks the New York–Vermont border. The city's commercial future was ensured the day the first trainload of farm products left Burlington for Boston. The railroad had built a port at Burlington, which allowed all the lakeside farming communities to ship their produce first by boat to Burlington, and then by train to Boston. The village grew into a town. Business flourished, and the town became a city.

But with the decline of the railroads, Burlington's port area decayed. The city itself, by then the home of the state's university, continued to thrive, but the area around the docks was a no-man's land, a virtual monstrosity, despite its ultra-scenic waterside location.

All that's changed today for the better. Since the 1960s, the city and the railroad have jointly cleaned up the dock area and transformed the lakeshore into attractive city parkland. Working together, business and government created the Waterfront Park and Promenade. In tandem, they also paved over much of the railroad bed that runs beside the lake and up onto the cliffs above the water.

The result is an attractive bike path which provides nearly continuous views of the lake and the distant islands.

The Bike Path:

Seven waterfront parks are strung out along the lakeshore. This path takes you to all of them, including a few with some terrific beach and swimming opportunities.

You'll begin at Oakledge Park. Be sure to visit the oak that sits on the ledge over the water in this park. This huge old tree has a plaque which explains that the tree was alive and thriving at the time of the signing of the Declaration of Independence. Standing by the oak, you'll look out across the lake to see the Burlington skyline to the north. Oakledge Park has plenty of picnic tables, some good swimming, and several private, hidden ledges where you can sit peacefully and look out across the windy lake.

Heading north from Oakledge, you'll follow the shoreline closely for most of the ride. If you look west, you can see the distant blue peaks of the Adirondacks across miles of lake water. If you look east, you'll sometimes see houses and industrial buildings, but you'll quite often see fields and extensive stands of sturdy hardwoods.

North of Oakledge Park, the bikeway briefly travels over some very quiet side streets and then returns to the shoreline. It's easy to lose your way here. The signage is poor. If you can't find where to go, look for the railroad bed. The path is adjacent to the railroad.

Next you'll ride through the renovated Waterfront Park and Promenade. After that comes a slight hill. At the top of the hill the path continues to follow the shoreline, but at cliff height, so your views of the lake and its islands are spectacular. Biking along this segment, you'll pass the public beaches, with very pleasant swimming areas.

The bikeway ends at the mouth of the Winooski River, a small peaceful river that'll make you wish for a canoe.

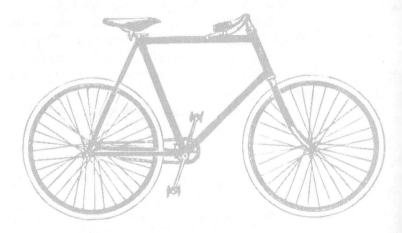

Food Facilities Nearby: A few restaurants in the city; prime picnic spots in the parks and on the ledges high above the lake.

Restrooms: In the parks, May to October.

Special Precautions: The winds from Lake Champlain can be very, very strong.

Best Parking Lot: Oakledge Park.

Directions: From I-89, take the Route 2 exit that leads into Burlington. Route 2 becomes Main Street, which descends down a long and steep hill toward Lake Champlain. Near the bottom of the hill, turn left onto Pine Street, and then right onto Flynn. You will see signs at this turn which point toward Oakledge Park.

For More Information: The Burlington Parks and Recreation Department, 216 Leddy Park Road, Burlington, Vermont 05401. Tel: (802) 864-0123.

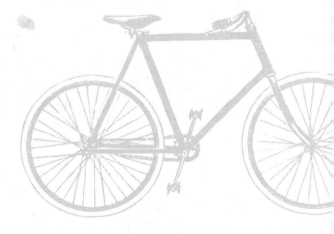

3. The South Burlington Recreation Path

SOUTH BURLINGTON, VERMONT

General Description:

A spider web of about 6 miles of recreation path, spinning out like spokes in a wheel from a public park in the center of this bustling city.

Level of Difficulty: Average to challenging; on-street biking in a few spots.

Type of Scenery: A scenic overlook; some forested areas and wetlands; some very urban biking on busy city streets.

Condition of Pavement: Good.

General Background:

The people of South Burlington began weaving this spider web of recreation paths in the late 1980s, when a citizens' group came up with the idea of recreation paths to link the city's schools and parks. Through an informal survey, city officials learned that taxpayers would fund the project. Development plans were submitted to an enthusiastic city council and other agencies, and the work began.

This is a recreation path with a motto: "A Green Ribbon to tie South Burlington together." The path does just that. By the mid 1990s, the strands of the spider web had been woven through almost every South Burlington neighborhood. Eventually, these paths will connect with those of Burlington.

The Bike Path:

Like a spider web, this recreation system really has no beginning or end. You just get on and ride. The strands loop all through the town, but most of them do return, one way or another, to Dorset Street Park, a new 65-acre park near the city's geographical center.

Cyclists can ride out of that park on off-road paved paths in northerly, southerly, and westerly directions. In Dorset Street Park and in another, smaller park, Farrell Park, 2 large maps picture the complete system.

Although this path is designed for commuting, there are some lovely views. If you ride south from Dorset Street Park, you'll see the distant Green Mountains, Mount Mansfield, and Camel's Hump. If you ride west, toward Shelburne Road, you'll briefly leave the very busy traffic behind as the path disappears completely into woods and pasturage. One leg of this path brings you to Overlook Park, a scenic overlook with a fantastic view of Lake Champlain and the Adirondack Mountains.

Food Facilities Nearby: Many sandwich shops and restaurants in this urban area.
Restrooms: Dorset Street Park, May to October.
Special Precautions: This recreation path requires crossing several very busy highways; in a few places you must ride on streets, intermingling with fairly heavy traffic.
Best Parking Lot: Dorset Street Park.

Directions: To get to Dorset Street Park from Interstate 89, take Exit 14 East, the South Burlington exit. This is Williston Road. Near the Howard Johnson's, turn right onto Dorset Street and head south past the South Burlington High School and the city office building. Pass through several traffic lights to the confluence of three roadways: Dorset Street, Kennedy Drive, and Interstate 189 (not to be confused with 89). Head under the I-189 bridge, still following Dorset Street. Head up the hill. The Dorset Street Park is on the left. Take the first left at the intersection of Dorset Street and the Swift Street Extension.

For More Information: The South Burlington Recreation Department, 575 Dorset Street, South Burlington, Vermont 05403. Tel.: (802) 658-7956.

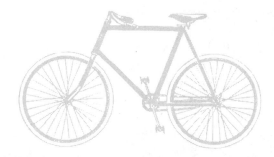

4. The Causeway Park Recreation Path

General Description:

A 4.1-mile flat path along an old railroad causeway that extends several miles across Lake Champlain.

Level of Difficulty: Easy.

Type of Scenery: Parkland; wetlands; Lake Champlain, with its distant islands and the far-off Adirondack Mountains of New York.

Condition of Pavement: Very fine gravel for much of the ride. Rough railroad ballast, uncomfortable for any but all-terrain bicycles, on the segment extending farthest into the lake.

General Background

In the last century, the Rutland Railroad carried farm products and city-bound passengers from Grand Isle, in the middle of Lake Champlain, over to Colchester, just north of Burlington. When the railroad was no longer used, the 2.8-mile causeway deteriorated. Ultimately, a western segment was demolished so ships could pass through more easily. It was no longer possible to walk across the water of Lake Champlain to get from Vermont to upstate New York.

The town of Colchester bought the causeway's decayed remains in the 1960s, but let it lie buried in overgrowth until the early 1990s, when townsfolk raised money to transform it into this unique recreation area.

Causeway Park opened to the public in 1994. Currently the path is gravel and ballast, but much of it is comfortable biking; officials hope one day to have enough money to pave its surface. Colchester citizens hope that one day their path will connect with the Burlington Bikeway (see separate entry), which runs along the shore of Lake Champlain just to the south. Both these paths, in fact, were once segments of the same railroad. Causeway Park begins just north of the mouth of the Winooski River; the Burlington Bikeway ends at the southern bank.

Cycling enthusiasts hope both paths will eventually become part of a much longer bikeway extending deep into Canada. Also on the wish list (but unlikely to materialize soon) is a lake ferry to meet cyclists at the end of the Colchester causeway and carry them to South Hero on Grand Isle.

Currently, the path's first 2 miles, from its start in Airport Park to the causeway's first bridge, are covered with fine gravel, quite comfortable to most cyclists and suitable for most bikes. The next 2.1 miles are covered with rough ballast. Town officials hope to improve this ballast with finer gravel in the near future, as soon as enough donations are raised.

The Bike Path:

This recreation path begins at Airport Park, in the town's western quadrant, and runs through Colchester

Bog, a natural area maintained by the University of Vermont. Next the path runs across a short stretch of private land and out onto the railroad causeway. The mostly rural path crosses only one road, a dirt road, for the whole of its length.

The causeway itself is built out of huge slabs of marble—the cheapest material then available. With a foundation like that, it has easily withstood a century of wind and water. Construction workers had to clean up the overgrowth that had covered the path after decades of disuse, but they found that the structure underneath remained strong.

Cycling to the end of the fine gravel will take you past Law Island, in Lake Champlain, to a stop where you'll be surrounded by mountain panoramas—great views of the Green Mountains in one direction, equally great views of the blue Adirondacks in the other. Photographers will want to spend a lot of time here.

The last 2 miles of the causeway are covered with original railroad ballast, a very rough ride. Many people leave their bikes and walk to the end. Fishermen say this is a great place to catch the best lake trout. The causeway ends where there used to be a turning bridge for the railroad, a necessity then (as it would be now) because of the heavy boat traffic on the lake.

Food Facilities Nearby: None.

Restrooms: At Airport Park in season. Open from May through September.

Special Precautions: Be careful of the weather. The causeway is exposed to the winds and changeable lake weather. Check out the weather report before you get caught in a storm.

Remember: if you are biking with the winds on your way out, you will be biking against them on your way back. Don't underestimate their power. Strong winds can make 4 miles feel like 8. The middle of the lake is often the windiest; winds generally come from the northeast.

Best Parking Lot: At Airport Park.

Directions: Take Exit 16 from Interstate 89 and head north on Route 2. At the fourth stoplight, turn left onto Blakely Road (Route 127), and head toward Malletts Bay. Continue heading west along Route 127, straight through one set of traffic lights at Bayside Park. Continue along this same road as it passes by a small section of commercial shops and a rural residential area. Route 127 turns off to the left; you continue straight to a stop sign at a 4-way intersection with Porters Point Road. Cross over Porters Point Road onto Airport Road and continue about a half-mile. Airport Park will be on your right.

For More Information: Colchester Parks and Recreation, P.O. Box 55, Colchester, Vermont 05446. Tel.: (802) 655-0811.

5. Franconia Notch State Park Recreation Path

General Description:

A 9.5-mile path winding through a spectacular mountain region, a nineteenth-century summer haunt for the world's rich and famous.

Level of Difficulty: Very challenging; rippling undulations, steep climbs and descents; a definite overall downhill slope from north to south.

Type of Scenery: Every well-known site in Franconia Notch: natural gorges and numerous waterfalls, swimming and fishing lakes, wooden walking bridges over mountain streams, the Cannon Mountain Aerial Tramway.

Condition of Pavement: Good.

General Background:

This is one of New England's most exciting bike paths, yet, oddly, it's also one of New Hampshire's best-kept secrets.

It's hard to understand why. There *is* no better way to see this crowded state park than from the seat of a bicycle. While others parade in cars along the 2-lane highway at 45 miles per hour, trying to catch a glimpse of natural beauty amidst the speeding semis, the recreation-path cyclist can stop whenever the urge strikes, smell the wildflowers, and enjoy the scenery. Despite this, the Franconia Notch recreation path is little used by cyclists, compared with the region's other major paths.

There are probably several reasons for this. The path is a bit too difficult for young children, or for adults who are not quite in condition. We saw several couples who had started out intending to ride the length of the path but gave up after the first several miles riding north. Another reason could be the history of Franconia Notch and the unusual story behind the construction of the recreation path itself.

For well over a century, the natural spectacles in the Notch—the crystal-clear lakes, the rushing streams, the peaceful deciduous forests of birch and ash and maple— have drawn summer visitors from around the world. In the mid-1940s, federal highway engineers decided that the 2-lane road through the Notch ought to be widened into an interstate highway. Locals were dismayed. Environmental groups fought back, delaying development for years and claiming that a wider highway would threaten the ecological stability of the region.

The thwarted engineers compromised. Through a special act of Congress, the Franconia Notch stretch of I-93 became a 2-lane interstate. Rather than build a 4-lane road, highway designers made the existing road safer and built better parking and viewing areas.

And—they built the recreation path. The new path parallels the highway, sometimes closely and sometimes at

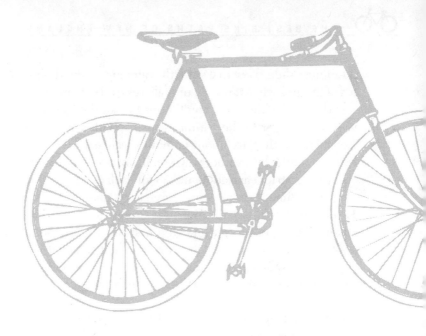

a distance. Designers have routed the path so recreationists can visit each scenic attraction.

The Bike Path:

For a full experience, you'll want to stop at the various
sights along the way, lock your bikes, and walk to the
waterfalls or ride the tram to the mountaintop. Bring bike
locks and a picnic. Plan on devoting a full day to this 9-mile
path.

If you plan on an out-and-back ride of 18 miles, we
suggest you begin at the southern end of the bike path, at
the Flume parking area. At the Visitor Center is a free

20-minute slide show that's worth watching, and old photos of the area when it was an upscale resort destination.

If you have the time, you'll want to visit the Flume, a waterfall. To get to the Flume, you may either walk the Loop Trail to the site (about an hour's walk each way), or ride the shuttle bus. Either way, you'll have to pay. In 1995, the fee was $6 for each adult and $3 for each child.

The Flume is an immense gorge at the base of Mount Liberty that was cut through the granite by cascading water. The European settlers who first saw the Flume in 1808 recognized it immediately as an area of great natural beauty. The walking paths in the area are also particularly pretty. One long covered bridge for walkers crosses a deep gorge.

After biking north from the Flume along the recreation path for more than a mile, you'll come to site called the Basin—a waterfall with a pothole-like pond at its base, bored out of the granite.

About halfway along the path's length, you'll come to the campground. This area is also a keystone in the state park's hiking-trail system. Four important trails set out from the valley at this point, climbing both valley walls. The Lonesome Lake trail—leading to Lonesome Lake, much higher up in the mountains—is particularly popular.

Several miles north of the campground are a pair of famous attractions: the Old Man of the Mountains, a natural rock formation 1,200 feet above the valley floor, also called "The Great Stone Face" in the writings of Nathaniel Hawthorne and Daniel Webster. Below the Old Man is Profile Lake, a crystal-clear lake said to reflect the Old Man's profile, although we did not see it. Profile Lake has some great trout fishing. Canoes are welcomed, but swimming is forbidden.

Toward the end of the recreation path, you'll come to the Cannon Mountain parking area. You can take a tram up the mountain ($8 for each adult; $4 for each child) or you can walk up the trail. The trail is steep (Cannon Mountain is 4,200 feet above sea level) and will require at least an hour's walking each way.

Continuing north along the recreation path, past Cannon Mountain, you'll find Echo Lake, a perfect place to stop and swim after a hot bike ride. After a rest, you can return to the Flume, biking back down the recreation path. You'll do more coasting on the way back, but you'll still have to pedal in places.

The path doesn't end at Echo Lake, although most people seem to stop here. The final segment continues into the White Mountain National Forest to hook up with 2 hiking trails. This segment crosses the Skookumchuck Brook via an old highway bridge closed to motorized traffic. There are some great photo opportunities here.

The last mile of the trail, continuing north from the bridge, is a gentle but persistent downhill ride through beautiful open fields. If you ride here in the middle of June, you'll ride through fields painted purple, white, and rose by the lupine that bloom here.

Food Facilities Nearby: The Flume Visitor Center, Cannon Mountain parking lot. The Summit House, on top of Cannon Mountain, serves lunch. (These are called "cafeterias," which tells you what you need to know about the food.)

There are numerous picnic areas and scenic spots where you can stop, sit, and enjoy your own picnic lunch.

Restrooms: The Flume Visitor Center, the Basin East, the Basin West, Lafayette Campground, the Old Man parking lot, Cannon Mountain parking lot, on top of Cannon Mountain.

Special Precautions: This recreation path requires a relatively high degree of fitness. If you're not sure you can do 18 miles of hilly biking in one day, you might arrange for a pickup.

This path has a posted speed limit of 20 miles per hour! Park officers say the north-to-south drop allows cyclists to build up to speeds which become seriously dangerous.

Officials ask cyclists to (1) obey the posted limit, (2) wear helmets, (3) walk through all parking lots, (4) travel single file, and (5) watch out for the children, elderly, and walkers who are also invited to use this recreation path. There have been several serious accidents on this path. Cyclists who want to travel at high speeds should use automobile roads and not the recreation path, park officials warn.

Many bike paths in New England allow in-line skating. This one does not.

Best Parking Lot: To bike round-trip on the recreation path, park at the Flume Visitor Center parking lot, at the park's southern end. There should be ample parking here on all but the busiest days.

To bike the recreation path in the north-to-south direction only, park at Echo Lake or Cannon Mountain. Since Echo Lake has a swimming beach, this parking area gets crowded on hot days.

Directions: For all parking areas, follow signs from Interstate 93, the Franconia Notch Parkway. You can also get to the Flume Visitor Center from Route 3, and to the Echo Lake parking area from Route 18.

For More Information: Franconia Notch State Park, Franconia, New Hampshire 03580. Tel.: (603) 823-5563.

Or: The New Hampshire Department of Resources and Economic Development, Division of Parks and Recreation, Box 856C, Concord, New Hampshire 03301. Tel.: (603) 271-3254.

Or: The White Mountain National Forest, Forest Supervisor, Box 638, Laconia, New Hampshire 03247. Tel.: (603) 528-8721.

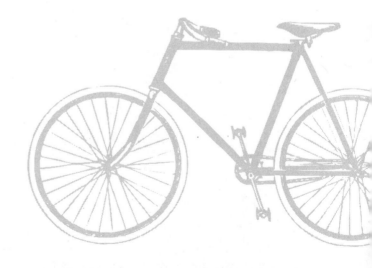

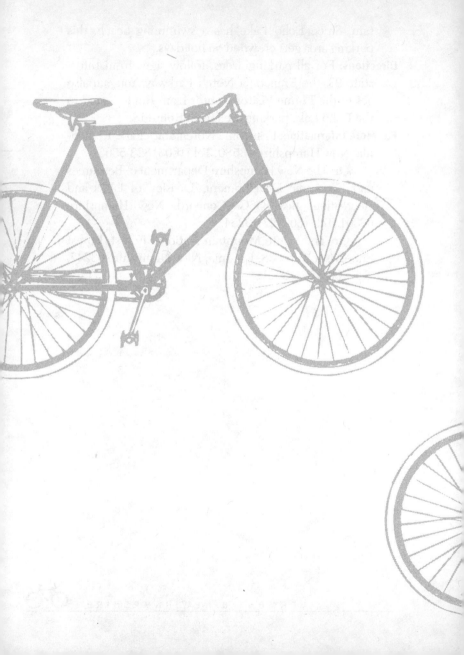

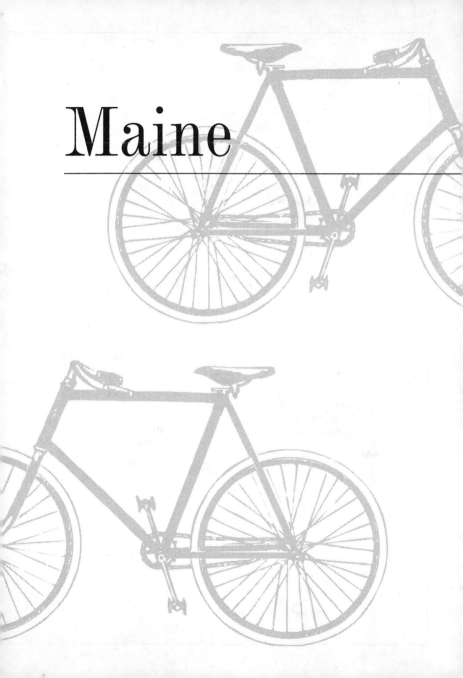

Maine

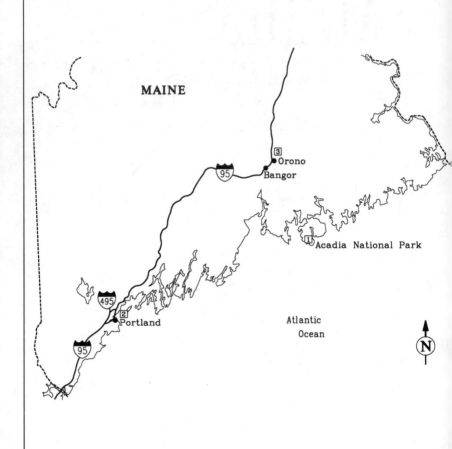

Maine

1. The Carriage Paths of Acadia National Park

MOUNT DESERT ISLAND, MAINE

General Description:

About 44 miles of interlaced roads and paths, closed to motor vehicles, wind through this visually spectacular national park.

Level of Difficulty: Very easy to very challenging; something for everyone.

Type of Scenery: Shangri-La! Awe-inspiring cliff-height views of the islands in Frenchman Bay; 17 incredible granite bridges, each individually designed; miles of shoreline; numerous freshwater lakes; bald mountains of granite formed during the last glacial period; endless forests of conifer and hardwood; majestic coastline views and peaceful rides through deep aromatic forests, far away from traffic and crowds.

Condition of Pavement: All roads are gravel-covered, but surfaces vary from fine cinder that's comfortable for all bikes, to deep and rutted gravel navigable only by mountain bikes.

General Background:

If you can bike only one path in New England—choose Acadia National Park!

Nothing like these carriage roads exists anywhere else in the world. In the late 1800s, when many of the world's fabulously wealthy families built mansions at Newport, a few more independent families summered on Mount Desert Island. Among these were the Rockefellers. Beginning in the early 1900s, John D. Rockefeller, Jr., scion of the oil baron, began covering his island estate with these roads, so his visitors could enjoy the rugged mountains and jagged coastline from the seat of an elegant horse-drawn carriage.

Acadia, the only national park to have been donated entirely by private citizens, was begun in 1919; President Woodrow Wilson signed a bill making it the first national park east of the Mississippi River. Since then, the park has grown as more families have contributed land; today it has 35,000 acres.

After the land was donated, Rockefeller remained commited to his roads. He built 57 miles in total, until they led to all the most inspiring vistas on the island. And he continued to maintain what he built, employing a 100-man work crew whose sole responsibility was carriage-road maintenance.

When Rockefeller died in 1960, the family handed the maintenance responsibilities over to the federal government. Federal officials, hampered by lack of funding, did very little. The roads began to fall apart. Vegetation grew so thickly that in many places the 16-foot-wide roads narrowed to 6 or 7 feet of navigable pathway. Culverts and ditches filled with detritus, causing washouts. The finely graded crowns eroded, leaving only large foundation stones.

In 1991, David Rockefeller and the Friends of Acadia, a citizens' group, proposed a plan for rehabilitation that was accepted by the park service. The government would supply the $4 million needed to bring the roads back to the level maintained by John Jr. In turn, the citizens' group would raise $4 million from private donations to be put in trust. Income from the trust would pay for maintenance.

Work began to bring these roads back up to the Rockefeller standard. Friends of Acadia have yet to raise the full $4 million, but they have received donations from several large benefactors and hope to make up the rest from small, individual gifts. A donation of $17.50 buys maintenance-in-perpetuity of 1 foot of carriage road.

The Bike Paths:

By now, most of the roads have been improved. Their surfaces are often smooth enough to allow access to most types of bikes; in a few places the pedaling is still rather rough.

When planning rides, allow plenty of time to stop and look at the granite bridges. Each was individually designed to blend with the surrounding cliffs and ponds. Some bridge enthusiasts plan their ride as a tour of the most spectacular of these creations.

The park has a special carriage-road map available, which you must have when you set out for the day. Intersections are numbered on the maps. On the roads, at each intersection, you will find signposts with these numbers. By matching the numbers on the signposts to the numbers on your map, you'll find out where you are. This can be crucial if you're at the end of a cycling day and you come across a signpost that points toward Eagle Lake in one direction, and Eagle Lake in the other direction. (This really happens at one intersection.) Which is the shortest route? Without the map, you can't tell.

Included here are descriptions of 4 loop rides, ranging from very easy to very difficult. They are described in terms of the numbered intersections.

Ride 1: The Eagle Lake Loop. This 6.1-mile ride, very easy, loops around the lake. There are several scenic vistas. Begin at the Eagle Lake parking lot, near Intersection 9, and head around the lake to Intersection 8, then 7, then back to 9. The ride should take less than an hour, if you don't make any stops. But you'll want to make lots of stops, so allow more time. This is a great place for young children or for people towing infants. The road is very finely graded and is quite smooth. It is also the most popular of the paths for biking. Expect crowding on summer days. Go early, or expect to have difficulty finding a parking spot.

Ride 2: The Witch Hole Pond Figure-Eight. Some people begin this ride from the Visitor Center parking lot, near Intersection 1. We don't recommend that. The path from the parking lot to Intersection 1 is very steep, accessible only to the strongest of cyclists with mountain bikes. Rangers say many accidents occur here.

We suggest you begin at the Eagle Lake parking area, at Intersection 6. From 6 to 4 is a little more than a mile in distance. The Witch Hole Pond Figure-Eight double-loop, from 4 to 5 to 3 to 2 to 1 to 3 to 2 to 4, is about 4.4 miles. By biking back and forth between 4 and 6, you'll add another 2 miles; the distance will be about 6.5 miles. Park staff say this is probably the easiest loop ride, with only a few short

5-percent grades. These roads are also covered with very fine, well-packed gravel, making them excellent for family rides and very popular. Arrive early on summer days.

Ride 3: Around-the-Mountain Loop. This ride of almost 14 miles, also out of the Eagle Lake parking area, is for cyclists who want a good workout on steeper and rougher roads. One ranger describes this as his favorite after-work ride. He strings the intersections this way: 6 to 8 to 10 to 12 to 19 to 20 to 21 to 14 to 10 to 8, then either back to 6, or to 7 and then 6, taking the long way around Eagle Lake. The rise between Intersections 10 and 12 is about 300 feet, so steep that Rockefeller engineered several switchbacks, very rare in this road network.

This road is difficult, but many people think you'll see the best scenery in the park from these vistas. You're above the treeline in places, so you'll see views of Somes Sound, Eagle Lake, and even Frenchman Bay. On a clear day you can see Camden, 70 miles away. This loop includes 7 of the 17 stone bridges Rockefeller built, including Hemlock Bridge, Waterfall Bridge, and Amphitheater Bridge, voted by park staff as the best place in the park to have a picnic.

Ride 4: The Day Mountain Loop. Intersections 37, 38, and 36. On paper, this looks like a good, short ride. Don't be fooled. This is a steep, rugged climb up a mountain, only for the most devoted of cyclists. Some of the park staff have never biked this carriage path, in part because it is used during the warm months by teams of workhorses pulling large wagonloads of tourists. The horses' hooves chop up the road, and cyclists have a hard time negotiating the holes.

Food Facilities Nearby: The Jordan Pond House, open in season, serves lunch, dinner, and afternoon tea on the lawn. You can get popovers and homemade ice cream, or you can order a full dinner. The restaurant is located at the intersection of the Park Loop Road and a carriage road, at the southern end of Jordan Pond.

Restrooms: Public restrooms are plentiful in the park, at the visitor centers, but not necessarily near the carriage roads. Some public restrooms are open May to October only; others are open year-round.

Special Precautions: Too many people set out to bike these extensive, deep-woods roads without adequate preparation, warn Acadia's park rangers. Cyclists should be sure to consider these points:

(1) These roads are extensively interlaced and can be confusing, even to those familiar with them. The park service has organized a system of numbered signposts that, when accompanied by park-service carriage-road maps pointing out the numbered signposts, keep most cyclists from becoming lost.

Carry your park-service carriage-road map with you. They are available from the wooden boxes at the following 7 signposts:

Signpost 6, at Eagle Lake
Eagle Lake boat-launch area
Bubble Pond
Jordan Pond stonepost gates
Signpost 17, the Day Mountain Bridge
Brown Mountain parking lot

(2) The elevation of the 17 mountains on the island vary from 200 to 1,500 feet above sea level.

Though the elevation of the carriage roads is obviously not that extreme, some climbs are considerably steeper than others. If you have young or beginning cyclists in your group, park rangers suggest that you start with the Eagle Lake or Witch Hole Pond circuit. If you decide to try other carriage roads, find out about their elevations first.

(3) Even in the summer, weather and temperatures can vary considerably. Dress in layers. Summer temperatures range from 45 to 85 degrees; spring and fall temperatures, from 30 to 70 degrees. Watch out for black flies during May and June.

(4) Bring liquids. Bring quick-energy snacks to recover from sudden energy depletions.

(5) Some cycling brochures suggest you also bike the automobile roads, including the scenic Park Loop Road. Mount Desert Island is the second-most-visited of our national parks. If you choose to bike that road during the summer season, be aware that traffic is very, very heavy. Part of the Loop Road is one-way and two-lane, but the two-way section of the Loop Road is very narrow and can be quite dangerous.

(6) The small section of carriage roads at the southern end of the island, outside the park boundaries, is for horses. The horses' hooves dig up the roads so much that cyclists have a difficult time on them. Leave those paths for the horses, and stay within the park's boundaries.

Horses are allowed on some carriage-path roads in the national park. When you see horses, stop and let them pass by, as a courtesy. Bikes always yield to horses.

(7) No matter how many times rangers warn mountain bikes off the hiking paths, some cyclists just don't listen. One ranger told us she found a fellow who had carried his mountain bike all the way up to the top of one of the steepest hiking trails, a trail that included many ladder sections. *Please don't do this.* Cyclists who use hiking trails which are clearly forbidden to bikes ruin things for everyone.

Best Parking Lot: The Eagle Lake parking lot fills up very early in the morning on summer days. By afternoon, the circuit around the lake is a mob scene. Go very early, if this is where you want to park.

The Hulls Cove parking lot at the Visitor Center has more room, but the path to Witch Hole Pond is quite steep. Most cyclists will have to walk their bikes up parts of this path. Rangers recommend that cyclists not use the path.

Jordan Pond is a very popular parking area. There are several different sites; parking is usually possible.

The least-used parking lots are at Parkman Mountain and Brown Mountain, both located on Routes 3 and 198. The Park Loop Road does not come near this area; consequently, there are fewer visitors.

Directions: Take Route 3 from Ellsworth. To get to the Hulls Cove Visitor Center, veer off to the left along Route 3 once you cross the bridge onto the island.

To get to the Parkman Mountain and Brown Mountain parking lots, veer to the right on Routes 103 and 198. When the 2 roads separate at the head of Somes Sound (said to be the only true fjord on the Atlantic Coast), take the left fork and head south along

Route 198. Look for parking signs. (Don't be concerned when this road actually becomes Route 3 again.)

The Thompson Island information center, at the south end of the Route 3 bridge onto the island, is open during the warmer months. You can find park-service maps and other information here, to get started.

The park's winter headquarters is located along Route 233 near Eagle Lake. To get there from the Route 3 bridge, veer right along Route 102/198; take a left on Route 198 at the head of Somes Sound and then a quick left on Route 233. The headquarters building will be on your right.

For More Information: Superintendent, Acadia National Park, P.O. Box 177, Bar Harbor, Maine 04609. Tel.: (207) 288-3338.

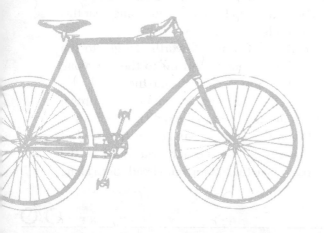

2. The Back Cove Recreation Path

General Description:

A 3.5-mile flat path around a saltwater cove just north of the city center. About 5.5 miles will be completed by the end of 1996.

Level of Difficulty: Very easy.

Type of Scenery: Wildlife sanctuary; marine waterfowl; marshland; the city skyline.

Condition of Pavement: Very fine stone dust, comfortable for all bikes.

General Background:

The Back Cove Park is part of the park system designed in 1905 by Frederick Law Olmsted's firm, the same firm that designed the parks of Boston and New York City. The Olmsted firm suggested that Portland create a string of parks that included the Eastern Promenade, a high cliff overlooking the islands of Casco Bay. Olmsted also designed the Back Cove Park, near the promenade.

The Portland citizenry thought Olmsted was crazy. In those days, the Back Cove, a saltwater inlet with a very narrow opening to the sea, was a disgusting cesspool at the center of Portland's casually organized waste-disposal system.

But the city's mayor, James P. Baxter (son of Governor Percival Baxter who created Maine's famous Baxter State Park), wanted to go ahead with Olmsted's plan. Baxter bought the Back Cove with city tax dollars.

This action was considered frivolous by the city's voting population. Baxter lost the next election. Unfazed by this electoral reprimand, Baxter ran in the next election, won, and returned to his park project. However, he could not cajole the voters into funding a city park. The cove continued to smell of sewage until about 1960.

Water clean-up efforts began in that decade, but the park itself wasn't built until the 1980s. In 1985, the city funded the first 2 miles of the recreation trail around the water; when the highway bridge over the inlet was rebuilt in 1989, a bikeway/walkway was added. The Back Cove recreation circuit was complete.

By the 1990s, building recreation paths had become a

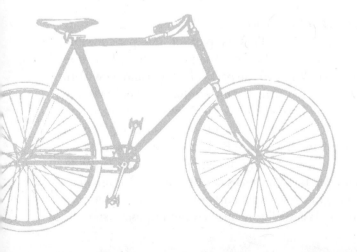

mini-craze in Portland. By 1996, the city hopes to have completed another 2 miles, paved this time. The new section will begin at the Back Cove Recreation Path, near the southern end of the Washington Avenue bridge (also called Tukey's Bridge), and will extend through the Eastern Promenade. Portions of the path will be 12 to 14 feet wide. The path, linking the Back Cove with the city's waterfront, will snake along the high cliffs of the Eastern Promenade all the way to the city's busy downtown harbor, ending at the intersection of Franklin and Commercial Streets. When this is completed, the 5.5-mile recreation path will doubtless rank among the most interesting, most scenic, and most entertaining of urban bike paths.

The Bike Path:

This pretty path makes a complete loop around the Back Cove, a saltwater cove with an inlet so narrow that the cove is more like a pond. Now a wildlife sanctuary, the Back Cove is a favorite of wind surfers, whom we saw sailing on the coldest and windiest of fall days.

For kids, a special attraction is the ride over the cove's inlet on Tukey's Bridge—also the bridge for Interstate 295 and for Washington Avenue, a main city street leading into downtown Portland. Don't be afraid: the bike/pedestrian lane over the bridge is well separated from automobile traffic. Biking over the bridge is quite safe. Cyclists can even stop and enjoy the view from the center of the bridge.

The path was built for walkers and joggers as well as cyclists; emphasis is on recreation rather than speed. High-speed cyclists are asked to use automobile roads instead, except for the bike lane over Tukey's Bridge.

Food Facilities Nearby: None on the path; excellent restaurants a short drive away, along the revitalized city docks, near the Fore River and Casco Bay.

Restrooms: Portable toilets May to October, Preble Street parking lot.

Special Precautions: Watch out for wind. On a windy day the trip over the bridge may be a little intimidating. Some people walk their bikes, even though the bike/pedestrian path is safely separated from the automobile traffic.

This is a multi-purpose trail. City officials ask cyclists to be careful of pedestrians.

Best Parking Lot: Preble Street Park, Payson Park.

Directions: Take the Forest Avenue exit off Interstate 295, Exit 6A or 6B. Head north to the intersection of Forest Avenue and Baxter Boulevard. Turn right. The next intersection is Preble Street. Turn right to get to the Preble Street parking lot. Turn left and you will arrive at Payson Park.

For More Information: Division of Parks and Recreation City of Portland, 17 Arbor Street, Portland, Maine 04103. Tel.: (207) 874-8793.

3. The University of Maine at Orono Bike Path

General Description:

A flat path of 2.25 miles, extending from the University of Maine campus through a forest preserve to the village of Old Town on Marsh Island.

Level of Difficulty: Very easy.
Type of Scenery: Forest preserve; a large deer herd; cornfields; farming country.
Condition of Pavement: Excellent.

General Background:

One misty Sunday afternoon in the late fall, we came across 6 deer munching on the rich clover planted on both shoulders of this paved bike path. We watched; they chewed. It was like being in the middle of the painting *The Peaceable Kingdom*, and it stayed that way for a quarter-hour, until a jogger emerged from the woods and startled the animals. Only then, when the deer began running, did we see that there had been not 6 but 30 animals in this group; the others had stayed hidden in the forest.

We learned more about the deer herd later. The University of Maine at Orono, the main campus of the state university, sits on an island at the confluence of the Stillwater and Penobscot Rivers. Marsh Island is a game preserve; hunting is forbidden.

The deer may know this. As long as people approach quietly, the animals stand and graze, patiently tolerating the intrusion.

We are told that an albino stag and his offspring live among this herd, although we can't say we saw him ourselves.

The Bike Path:

This fun, short little path begins at the university campus, behind the athletic fields. It is partly recreation trail, partly rail trail. This is an old bike path, built with a federal grant provided back in 1978.

The paved path is actually the main path running through a forest owned by the university. From this central artery spin a variety of side trails, ranging from actual dirt roads (most of which forbid automobiles) to narrow walking and mountain-biking trails. This is, in fact, one of the few paved trails we've seen that encourages cyclists to leave the pavement and set off through the woods on the dirt.

If you begin the paved path at the university, you will very quickly reach a country road where there are absolutely no signs telling you where the path goes. The bike path jogs down the road to the right a short distance, then turns left off the road and heads into the forest again. When you come to a T intersection, turn right down this very straight, very flat, quite short rail trail. (This is where we saw the deer herd.)

The rail-trail segment is part of the Veazie Railroad bed, a narrow-gauge railroad, privately owned, which began in Bangor and led to Old Town. The section from the campus to the rail trail is 1.45 miles; along the rail trail to the street is .8 miles. Eventually, town and city officials hope that most of the old railroad bed, about 12 to 15 miles long, will be paved for cycling.

The forest path is actually connected to a bike route that begins in Orono, on Kelly Road and Main Street, and runs through the town of Orono to the main campus, along the side of the road.

Food Facilities Nearby: None.

Restrooms: None.

Special Precautions: None.

Best Parking Lot: The University of Maine campus, but see below.

Directions: Take Route 2 into the town of Orono. Turn onto College Avenue, which runs along the Stillwater River. There isn't really any "best" parking lot in the university. Parking for visitors depends very much on the time of day, the day of the week, and the season of the year. Official university policy requests that visitors first go to the Police and Safety Building at 166 College Avenue, where they can get a map of the campus and a parking permit.

For More Information: The Recreational Sports Office, Room 140, The University of Maine, 5747 Memorial Gym, Orono, Maine 04469-5747. Tel.: (207) 581-1081.

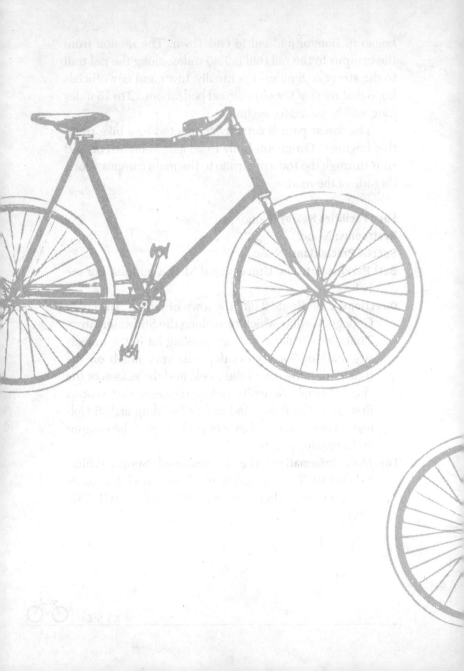

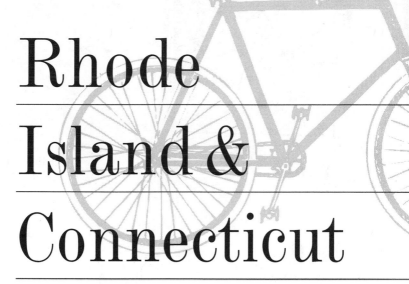

Rhode

Island &

Connecticut

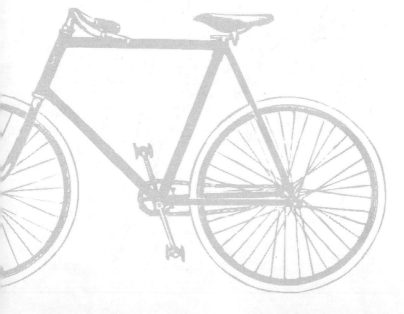

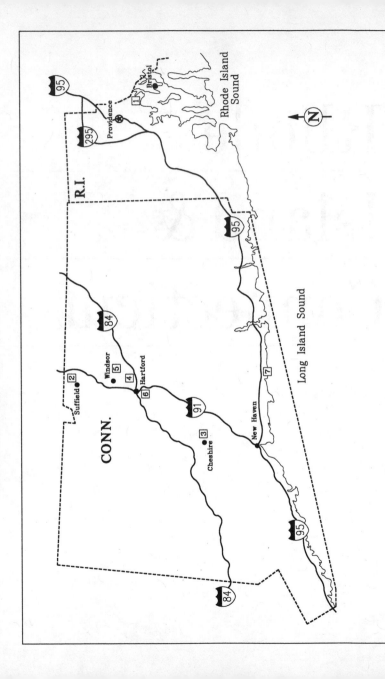

Rhode Island & Connecticut

1. The East Bay Bike Path

BRISTOL TO PROVIDENCE, RHODE ISLAND

General Description:

About 15 miles of mostly flat trail, through the enchanting coastal areas of Narragansett Bay, including the towns of Bristol, Warren, Barrington, East Providence, and Providence.

Level of Difficulty: Very easy.

Type of Scenery: Narragansett Bay shoreline; saltwater marsh with bird life; several river crossings; parklands; Rhode Island backyards; some urban cycling with a few stoplights; the last 2 miles include on-road biking.

Condition of Pavement: Excellent.

General Background:

This is quintessential New England! The path runs through surprisingly natural areas, considering the number of people who live on this bay.

The people of Rhode Island are particularly proud of their path, and it shows. In fact, many of those who most vehemently opposed the path's construction (and there were a lot) are now the East Bay Bike Path's proudest supporters. Neighbors who worried that the path would bring vandalism and petty theft now say the path's proximity is a selling point for their homes. Real-estate agents write "near the bike path" in sales brochures, often claiming that the path increases sales by thousands of dollars.

The path offers a tremendous variety of views, ranging from saltwater marshes and brackish rivers to the built-up industrialism of East Providence. It winds through 6 parks and passes near 2 more. On primo cycling days, 3,000 people bike here, a fact that has not been lost on local entrepreneurs. Sandwich shops and bike shops market their wares to the path's users, as do video stores, cleaners, groceries, and other stores—all of whom provide bike racks.

This path was designed for commuters to ride safely into Providence. All along the path, signs say: "Commuters welcome." In 1992, the fourth segment of the path, leading commuters from East Providence across the interstate bridge and into Providence, was opened. Some of this final segment is actually on automobile roads and is not particularly enjoyable for recreational cyclists.

The Bike Path:

Restaurants abound, beginning at the path's start, at Independence Park on Bristol Harbor, with its large flock of extremely expensive sail- and powerboats. The path runs through wetlands for about a mile to Colt State Park, where there are a number of recreational facilities, picnic areas, and restrooms.

From Colt State Park into Warren the ride is somewhat suburban, but there are plenty of views of marshes and tidal pools. The path is so well designed that cyclists don't have a sense of biking in a built-up area, although there are frequent road crossings. In Warren, cyclists cross busy roads.

After a brief ride along the town's main street, the path crosses a marshy area with 2 short bridges. Both bridges were railroad trestles which, by the time the path was built, were so decayed that they needed to be rebuilt. They are now covered with wooden planks discouraging high-speed cycling. The bridges are also favored as fishing spots.

The first of the 2 bridges, crossing the Palmer River, offers spectacular views of wetland wildlife. The next bridge crosses the Barrington River. Haines State Park lies on the Barrington–East Providence line.

Beginning in East Providence, the path becomes more urban, although it continues to travel along the coastal regions. At Crescent View Road in East Providence, consider taking a short detour to Carousel Park. Turn left onto Crescent View and bike about a quarter-mile toward the water. The huge carousel, listed on the register of historic

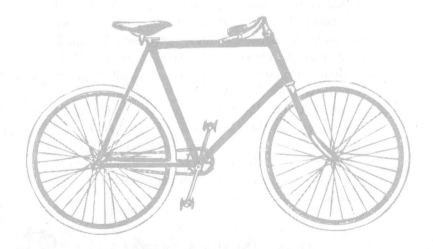

places, is obvious (you'll probably hear the music), but there's also a sign.

After the first 12 flat miles, there rises one hill, neither very long nor very steep, but annoying if you've grown used to an easy ride. At the top of the hill the path travels along a busy highway for about a mile, which is also annoying if you've grown used to biking without breathing exhaust fumes.

At the end of this mile is the Veterans Memorial Parkway parking lot. Below is the Providence River; beyond the river are the pink and green and white row houses of Providence.

After this parking lot, the path descends a hill into a very urban environment. For a short distance, you must bike on streets in traffic, then pick up a separate path. You cross the Providence River on the Washington Bridge on I-195, and end at India Point Park.

Food Facilities Nearby: An endless array of interesting-looking gourmet, deli, and sandwich places; several pizza and trendy outdoor restaurants; convenience stores in each town; if you hit it right at Colt State Park, on a Saturday or Sunday afternoon, you might be able to get a grilled hamburger or hotdog with soda at one of the kids' soccer games.

Restrooms: Colt State Park; Haines State Park; Carousel Park.

Special Precautions: This path, open to walkers, joggers, and skaters, will be crowded on weekends. Go early to beat the crowds. Cyclists have the right-of-way; walkers are welcome, but are responsible for moving out of the way of cyclists. (This is unusual trail protocol.) They are also asked to walk against cycling traffic, as they would on an automobile road.

The path crosses 49 roads. There are 2 traffic-signal intersections, at County Road in Barrington and Main Street (Route 114) in Warren. Both these roads are heavily traveled.

Best Parking Lot: There are many good places to park, but we suggest you use the Independence Park lot or the Colt State Park lot in Bristol, or the Veterans Memorial Parkway lot in East Providence.

Directions: To Independence Park in Bristol, from Interstate 195: Take Exit 7 from the interstate, and head south on Route 114. Colt State Park is in Bristol, on 114. To reach the Independence Park lot, continue on 114 into the town's business district. At the road fork, Route 114 goes left. The parking lot is on the right.

To reach the Veterans Memorial Parkway parking lot, take the Riverside/East Providence exit from I-195 immediately to the east of the Washington Bridge on I-195. Head south on the parkway, following the signs to Riverside. On your right, near the beginning of this parkway, is the East Bay Bike Path parking facility, well marked.

For More Information: Colt State Park, Bristol, Rhode Island 02809. Tel.: (401) 253-7482.

2. The Windsor Locks Canal Towpath

General Description:

A 4.5-mile flat towpath along a berm that runs the length of the Windsor Locks Canal, along the Connecticut River.

Level of Difficulty: Very easy.

Type of Scenery: Mostly water and forest on both sides of the towpath; an aqueduct over Stony Brook's 10-feet-deep chasm; the ancient and eroding Enfield Dam; no automobile-road crossings.

Condition of Pavement: Cracked pavement with grass and weeds growing up. Repaving scheduled for completion by 1996.

General Background:

Across the continent, bike paths follow America's waterways. Wetlands, after all, are America's oldest transportation corridors.

But we suspect there is no other bike path quite like the one at the Windsor Locks Canal, where you bike most of the way along a raised berm, high above water on both sides.

Even more intriguing is the segment of towpath which becomes an aqueduct. Yes, we mean aqueduct as in "Roman aqueduct," where you and the water are carried up over another stream, in a kind of wooden "water-bridge." This was the solution to a complex problem posed to the canal's early engineers: how to make one stream of water cross over another stream of water without mixing up the flow. Engineers needed to solve this problem because, at one point, the old Windsor Locks Canal had to cross the deep Stony Brook, which flows into the Connecticut River by way of a 10-foot-deep chasm. Their creative aqueduct solution looks like today's common highway overpass, a wooden bridge allowing both the water and the towpath across the deep barrier.

The canal itself, dug to transport barges around a very shallow section of Connecticut River rapids, has long been out of use. The state has recently bought it and intends to develop it into a state park, with interpretive facilities and paved parking areas. The towpath will be made handicapped-accessible.

In the meantime, the property is open to the public.

The Bike Path:

Even in its deteriorated condition, this is one of the most popular recreation paths in the state. The towpath is used heavily during the warm months by walkers, joggers, and cyclists. It is closed to humans during the winter because of its popularity with bald eagles, who nest here to fish the shallow rapids when the rest of the river is frozen.

This is a rural ride. Pedaling along, you'll see farmlands, hardwood and pine forests, a few houses. The high

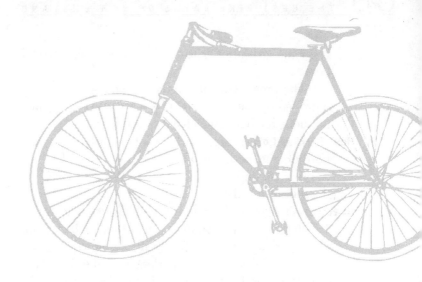

point is the aqueduct crossing. At the northern end is the Enfield Dam, once famous for its shad fishing derbies. The old dam has fallen apart but remains a popular fishing spot.

The canal's southern end, in Windsor Locks, begins in a somewhat industrialized area. We suggest you park in the more scenic northern-end parking lot in Suffield.

Food Facilities Nearby: None nearby. Picnic tables at the parking area at the northern end of the canal.

Restrooms: None as yet; the state intends to improve this situation.

Special Precautions: This area is closed to all human traffic from November through April. State officials and local residents give priority to the bald eagles who winter here.

This area is currently unimproved and not usually patrolled by state officials. There is no protective railing along the berm, which has steep slopes.

Best Parking Lot: A large parking lot in Suffield, at the northern end of the canal.

A small unpaved parking lot in Windsor Locks, at the southern end of the canal.

Directions: To get to the Suffield parking lot, take Route 159 into Suffield. Turn onto Canal Road, which leads to the parking lot, about .3 mile after the turn.

To the Windsor Locks parking lot, take Route 140 into Windsor Locks. Where Route 140 crosses the Connecticut River, on the east bank, you will see a row of factory buildings. Drive along the canal down to the end of this row of buildings, until a sign tells you motor vehicles are no longer allowed. People park here to use the towpath, although currently the parking lot is not state-run and, therefore, not patrolled.

For More Information: No contact phone number or address as yet. Check with the state's Department of Environmental Protection, Elm Street, Hartford, Connecticut 06106.

3. The Farmington Canal Linear Park

General Description:

A 2.8-mile, beautifully landscaped path, the first segment of a north-south 50-mile greenway that will stretch from New Haven to Northampton, Massachusetts.

Level of Difficulty: Very easy.

Type of Scenery: The Farmington Canal; a historic park featuring one of the locks that once operated along this long-defunct canal; semi-rural countryside.

Condition of Pavement: Excellent.

General Background:

The Farmington Canal, built by the industrialist Eli Whitney and several other businessmen, opened in 1828. Extending from New Haven Harbor north into Massachusetts, the 83-mile waterway, modeled after the eminently successful Erie Canal, was expected to boost the economies of the western Connecticut towns through which it ran. The canal's entrepreneurs in western Connecticut envied the success of Hartford, blessed with the Connecticut River. They hoped their human-made waterway would compete.

It did not. The 25-lock canal, never profitable, closed

in 1848. The right-of-way became a railroad, which *was* economically successful, operating with regular runs until 1982.

In concert with private groups, Connecticut state officials hope to turn the whole of this canal-cum-railroad into a biking-and-hiking greenway. If this happens, the Farmington Canal Greenway is likely to be New England's premier paved-path bike ride.

When the plan will come to fruition is anybody's guess, but solid steps have already been taken. Most of the right-of-way has been acquired. Construction of a section extending from the southern end of the existing Cheshire path and stretching several miles south toward New Haven may be completed in 1996, creating a contiguous path of 7 or 8 miles. Many of the greenway's segments are in the later planning stages. Look for much more to be done with this greenway within the next few years.

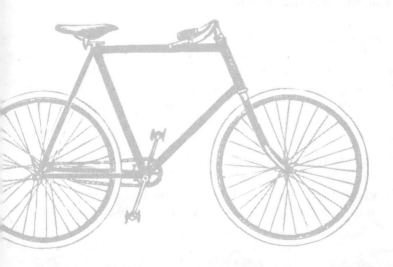

The Bike Path:

The upscale town of Cheshire, a short drive north from New Haven along Route 10, has the honor of having completed this greenway's first segment. The town's creation is exquisite: this little piece of bike-and-recreation path is beautifully landscaped. If other towns follow suit, New England will have a 50-mile path it can be proud of.

The people of Cheshire did not skimp. The path runs along what's left of the old waterway, which today flows along like a quiet country brook. Several attractively designed wooden bridges cross the brook at different points, so cyclists can look down into the flowing water. In places, attractive post-and-rail fencing, using wood to match the bridges, separates the public path from private property. All along the trail are benches of the same wood for weary travelers.

There are, as you might imagine, lots of people. This trail is a mecca for local families with young children. Expect lots of 4- and 5-year-olds learning to ride bikes on this trail, and scads of people of all ages learning to use in-line skates. This trail is also popular with joggers, walkers, and strollers, many of whom ignore the protocol of the 2-lane recreation path. Recreationists who want to move at any but the slowest speeds should plan to visit early in the morning.

Food Facilities Nearby: None.

Restrooms: None.

Special Precautions: This well-used but under-signed trail hosts recreationists who do not yet understand path protocol. We saw cyclists who rode on the left side of the pavement; 4-year-olds using inline skates with no parental supervision; walkers strolling 4 and 5 abreast. Do not expect to ride your bike here at normal speeds, unless you ride very early in the morning.

Best Parking Lot: Lock 12 Park, in the middle of the 2.8-mile path; Cornwall Avenue, at the northern end of the path.

Directions: This short section of path roughly parallels Route 10 through Cheshire. To get to Lock 12 Park from Route 10, turn west onto North Brooksvale Road and continue about a half-mile down into the valley.

To get to the Cornwall Avenue parking area off Route 10, turn west onto Cornwall Avenue and continue about a half-mile. The parking area is on your right.

For More Information: The Parks and Recreation Department, 559 South Main Street, Cheshire, Connecticut 06410. Tel.: (203) 272-2743.

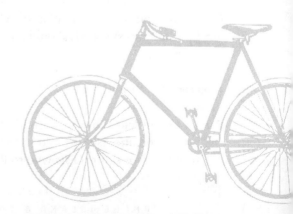

4. The Charter Oak Greenway

HARTFORD, EAST HARTFORD, AND MANCHESTER, CONNECTICUT

General Description:

A visionary greenway that will eventually lead from Hartford's Charter Oak Bridge to Bolton Notch State Park, more than 10 miles to the east.

Level of Difficulty: Average to very challenging.
Type of Scenery: Urban; interstate right-of-ways; parks and public lands; a short stretch on automobile roads.
Condition of Pavement: Excellent in some sections; other sections under construction.

General Background:

This extensive greenway, innovative for New England, is the result of federal transportation funds released for bike-path construction. Much of this particular greenway has been built along existing interstate right-of-way, but planners have provided very safe separation from the highway.

The state Department of Transportation is building this greenway in segments; the completed greenway will not be contiguous until near the end of the century. The strategy is simple: When the DoT rebuilds a highway within the greenway system, officials add in a separated bike-and-pedestrian path. In the short run, the piecemeal approach may seem a bit disorganized, but it seems to be the most effective way of bringing the whole bike system into existence as quickly as possible. And, indeed, the state has built many miles of bike path in an astonishingly short time. Despite this greenway's temporary fragmentation, we saw many cyclists, joggers, skaters, and walkers using the completed segments.

The Bike Path:

Four separate segments of path currently exist, with links to 2 other bike paths already completed. The path begins with a stretch of about a mile across the Charter Oak Bridge, with bike ramps at both ends of the bridge. Looking north from the center of the Charter Oak Bridge, you see the Hartford skyline and the Connecticut River, disappearing into the distance.

At the eastern end of the Charter Oak Bridge, you can take the bike ramp down to another path following the riverbank, built and managed by the non-profit agency Riverfront Recapture. (See separate entry.)

Currently there is a gap of about 1.5 miles in the Charter Oak Greenway itself. After descending from the bridge, cyclists must make their own way through city streets, riding in traffic, until the paved path starts again at Forbes Street, near I-84. A sign marks the beginning of this segment, but there is no parking lot. This 8-foot-wide segment—added in 1988, when the expressway was rebuilt—follows I-384 for a short period, passing Veteran's Memorial Park with its own bike-path spur. About a half-mile from the beginning of this segment, the Captain John Bissell Greenway branches off and heads north. (See separate entry.)

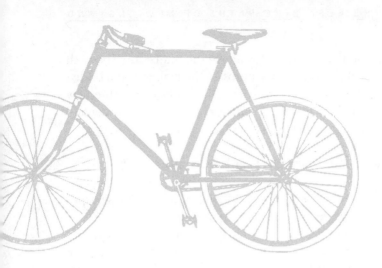

The Charter Oak greenway continues to Spencer Street in Manchester. Here the path crosses a busy street with a stoplight. Across the street, a newer section, 10 feet wide, breaks away from the I-384 right-of-way. It enters the Manchester Community Technical College campus, snaking among tall pines and around endless athletic fields. The path climbs a rather steep grade for a short distance.

Past the college, the greenway travels on-road for about .75 miles along designated bike lanes—Bidwell Street and Hartford Road—then goes off-road again, continuing along Hartford Road in a separated linear park.

Next the path becomes a kind of widened sidewalk along a road that bridges I-384, then climbs an embankment, so that the cyclist is above the interstate. The path ends at Route 83, where it crosses the highway on a bridge and enters Charter Oak Park. The distance from the new segment of the greenway, beginning at Spencer Street and extending to Charter Oak Park, is 3.9 miles.

Food Facilities Nearby: Not easily accessible.

Restrooms: None.

Special Precautions: Some difficult road crossings, especially at Spencer Street, require care.

A segment of .75 mile in on-road bike-lane cycling, along a somewhat heavily traveled road.

Best Parking Lot: Charter Oak Park in Manchester; Charter Oak Landing in Hartford; a commuter lot at Spencer Street; Veteran's Memorial Park.

Directions: Charter Oak Park is located at the intersection of Route 83 (Main Street) and I-384 (Exit 3). You will see signs for the park and for the bike path.

To get to Charter Oak Landing, the starting point for Charter Oak Greenway as well as the Riverfront recreation-path parking area, take the Brainard Road exit from I-91.

The commuter lot on Spencer Street is located near the I-384 expressway.

For More Information: The Bicycle-and-Pedestrian Coordinator, Connecticut Department of Transportation, 2800 Berlin Turnpike, P.O. Box 317546, Newington, Connecticut 06131-7546. No contact phone number.

5. The Captain John Bissell Greenway

General Description:

A 6-mile path, mostly off-road but with about 2 miles of on-road biking, that extends from the Captain John Bissell Bridge in Windsor to Manchester; intersects with the Charter Oak Greenway.

Level of Difficulty: Average.

Type of Scenery: The Connecticut River; some farmland; urban and suburban development; a nearby interstate highway.

Condition of Pavement: Excellent in some places; under construction in other places. Most of this greenway is paved-path, separated biking, but about 2 miles use automobile roads.

General Background:

The Captain John Bissell Greenway crosses the Bissell Bridge, follows the I-291 right-of-way, then enters the I-84 right-of-way. Connecticut transportation officials have adopted a somewhat unusual strategy of building bikeways along existing highway right-of-ways. This enables the speedy construction of some fairly extensive bikeway segments, since the time-consuming process of acquiring land isn't necessary.

The recreation cyclist's first reaction may be negative: biking near an expressway means the worst of road cycling, including racing trucks and breathing fumes. But for the most part, these bikeways do not hug the highways. The path may climb a ridge above the highway, or may veer off through parks or other public land, then return to the interstate right-of-way.

In urban situations, there are distinct advantages to this method of path construction. Besides enabling officials to avoid the lengthy and complex problem of land acquisition, these interstate right-of-ways help designers avoid some (but, alas, not all) dangerous road crossings. A

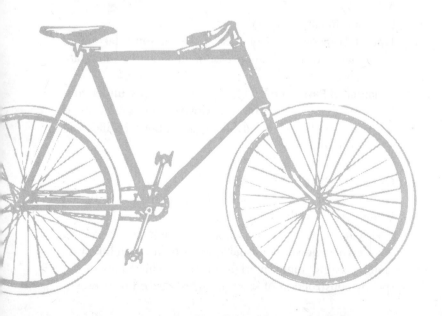

cyclist who wants to bike distances in an urban area will find the greenway system perfect.

But: we emphasize that in a few sections cyclists must ride on a road, competing for space with traffic, where planners have not been able to design a separate bike path.

The Bike Path:

The Captain John Bissell Greenway begins at the western end of the Captain John Bissell Bridge, at the state boat launch. This will eventually be the connecting point between the greenway and the Riverfront Recapture recreation path, expected to run along the Connecticut River's west bank. (See separate entry.)

Beginning at the state-boat-launch parking area, a bike-and-pedestrian ramp leads up onto the Captain John Bissell Bridge, with its own separated bike path. On the bridge's eastern end, an off-ramp lets the cyclist descend to Main Street in South Windsor. Here the greenway follows existing roadway rather than a bike path. Turn left onto Main Street, then right onto Chapel Street. After more than 2 miles of on-road biking, the path begins again at the Tolland Turnpike in Manchester, paralleling I-291. A short 5-percent grade climbs to a scenic overlook with a visibility of sometimes as much as 25 miles.

The path descends to Route 44 (where there is a spur into Wickham Park), then crosses that highway to begin another segment. This quite new 8-foot-wide segment follows I-84, briefly traveling along the Hockanum River. A specially built bike-path tunnel goes under I-84, climbs back to the surface again, then intersects with the Charter Oak Greenway. (See separate entry.) Turning right onto the Charter Oak Greenway takes you to Forbes Street, in the direction of Hartford; turning left takes you to Spencer Street, in the direction of Manchester and Bolton.

Food Facilities Nearby: Not easily accessible.

Restrooms: None.

Special Precautions: Connecticut's greenway system uses vehicular roadways. There are some on-road segments and several difficult road crossings at present.

This greenway is under construction. For the most up-to-date information, contact the bicycle coordinator at the address below.

Best Parking Lot: The state-boat-launch parking area, on the west bank of the Connecticut River.

Directions: From Route 159, take East Barber Street to the Connecticut River. The bike ramp will be on your left. The boat-launch parking area is below the Bissell Bridge.

For More Information: The Bicycle-and-Pedestrian Coordinator, Connecticut Department of Transportation, 2800 Berlin Turnpike, P.O. Box 317546, Newington, Connecticut 06131-7546. No contact phone number.

6. The Riverfront Recapture

General Description:

A 3.5-mile loop along both banks of the Connecticut River, crossing the river by way of 2 newly rebuilt bridges.

Level of Difficulty: Easy.

Type of Scenery: The best of downtown Hartford architecture; the city's system of beautifully designed waterfront parks; the scenic Connecticut River.

Condition of Pavement: Some sections just completed; some sections still under construction as of 1996. (See below.)

General Background:

Hartford is a city dominated by its river. The earliest European settlers arrived in this region by way of the river and wrested this expanse of the river's banks from the Indians who farmed and fished here. The tiny settlement grew into a thriving metropolis because of the river and eventually developed an important shipbuilding industry. Hartford even owes its insurance industry to the river, since its earliest insurance ventures grew out of the need to protect financially the ships launched by the city's industrialists.

Yet the river that nourished the city has also, on a yearly basis, threatened its existence. Each spring, the meltwater from the northern mountains inundates the

Connecticut. The river floods its low-lying banks and leaves behind thick layers of slippery silt.

In 1936, and then again in 1938, the flooding was severe. In response, the Army Corps of Engineers built huge dikes of concrete and of dirt for many miles up and down the river's banks. Hartford's dike stands 28 feet high, protecting the city effectively from flood, but also, quite effectively, separating the people from their river.

Because of these tall, ugly, and depressing barriers, it's easy to travel right through the center of Hartford, only a few feet from the river—without realizing the river exists. On a warm summer day, the people of Hartford cannot step out of their offices and homes and walk down along the water's edge.

In the 1980s, a non-profit alliance of the city's business leaders began to change that. They developed a fund-raising and revitalization program that, when completed, will give the river back to the people. The group's master plan calls for more than 6 miles of recreation path along both banks of the river. This walking-and-biking pathway, safely separated from vehicular traffic, will use 2 bridges that span the Connecticut: the Charter Oak Bridge and the Founders Bridge.

When the project is completed, cyclists will be able to ride a 3.5-mile loop across the Charter Oak Bridge, north along the east bank of the Connecticut River, across the Founders Bridge, and south again along the west bank of the Connecticut. On the west bank, the path will extend about 6 miles, from the Folly Brook Natural Area on Hartford's southern boundary to several miles north of the Captain John Bissell Bridge in Windsor.

In addition, the Riverfront recreation path will hook

into 2 separate bike-and-pedestrian systems built by the state's Department of Transportation: the Captain John Bissell Greenway and the Charter Oak Greenway. (See separate entries for both paths.)

When these 3 systems are completed, cyclists will be able to ride a 15-mile loop from the west bank of the Connecticut River, east on the Captain John Bissell Greenway to Manchester, and then west again on the Charter Oak Greenway back to the Riverfront recreation path. No other New England city has such an extensive network of interlaced bike paths.

The completion date for this visionary project is uncertain. Major segments are already finished; others are under construction; a few remain limited to the dream stage. Early plans called for completion of the 3.5-mile inner loop by 1996; now officials say it may be completed by 1997. Enough contiguous segments *are* complete, however, to make a short ride possible.

The Bike Path:

About two-thirds of the Riverfront Recapture's 3.5-mile loop is already ridable. If you park at Charter Oak Landing, you can bike north along the west bank of the Connecticut about halfway to Founders Bridge. Or you can bike up the bike ramp near the parking area and cross the Charter Oak Bridge to the river's east bank. The Charter Oak Bridge is also the Interstate 84 bridge, but the bikeway is safely separated from the traffic.

Crossing the Charter Oak Bridge, look north past the city skyline and see the wide Connecticut dissolve into the horizon. Descending from the bridge on another separated ramp, you can bike north along the river's east bank all the way to Founders Bridge. This bridge, leading into the center of Hartford, will be rebuilt to include a wide bike-and-pedestrian path in 1997. A promenade with grass and trees will lead back down to the Riverfront pathway.

To the north of Founders Bridge is the 88-acre Riverside Park, with its network of bike paths and walking paths snaking through the extensive lawns. It is not yet accessible from the bike path, but will be eventually.

Food Facilities Nearby: None.

Restrooms: Port-o-potties in the parks, during the summer months.

Special Precautions: The construction schedule is uncertain; check with Riverfront Recapture (information below). The organization also sponsors many river activities open to the general public.

This path, unprotected by the dike, is flooded each spring. The floods often leave a thick, slippery coating of silt which may make biking impossible. If you want to bike during early spring, check the path condition ahead of time. After flooding, it isn't safe to bike until the paths have been cleaned up.

Best Parking Lot: Charter Oak Landing in Hartford; Riverside Park in Hartford; Great River Park in East Hartford.

Directions: To Charter Oak Landing, from I-91, exit at Brainard Road; turn left at the ramp's end. Follow the River Boat signs.

To the Great River Park in East Hartford, take

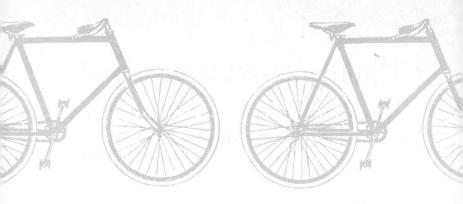

Pitkin Street east to East River Drive and turn left. Follow the signs to the boat launch.

For More Information: Riverfront Recapture, One Hartford Square West, Suite 104, Hartford, Connecticut 06106-1984. Tel.: (203) 293-0131.

7. Hammonasset Beach State Park

General Description:

A 1.2-mile stone-dust path winding along the park's coastline, with its extensive saltwater swimming beach.

Level of Difficulty: Very easy.

Type of Scenery: Saltwater beach; beachfront wetlands; developed park areas, picnic areas, and lots of ball fields.

Condition of Pavement: Stone dust. Comfortable for any bike, but not meant for high speeds.

General Background:

Located on a cove near the eastern end of Long Island Sound, this very popular family swimming area bustles during the summer. This means you'll find everything associated with a swimming beach located near a populated area: refreshment stands, first-aid buildings, acres of parking lots.

The state didn't initially intend to put a bike path into this park, but so many people brought bikes, drawn by the lure of biking along the coastline, that it became easier to build a bike path than to mediate conflicts between cyclists and motorists.

The stone-dust pathway extends from the parking area along the length of the swimming beach itself. This means you can bike a short distance along the path and leave behind the most crowded areas. Still, on a summer day you're unlikely to find peace and privacy.

The Bike Path:

The beginning of this bike path is difficult to find. It is marked with a small sign picturing a bike, which you will also see at a few other points along the path. The easiest way to find the path is to head toward the beach area from the parking area. If you park near the main pavilion, you'll find the path on the other side of the pavilion, nestled in between the building and the beach. Follow the stone-dust path along the beach, among stands of tall grasses, to the other end. From there, you can walk along some smaller paths that climb up into the rocks, where there is a viewing platform overlooking Long Island Sound's coastline and islands.

Food Facilities Nearby: During the summer months, plenty of hotdog-and-soda possibilities.

Restrooms: Summer only.

Special Precautions: Be sure to get there early on hot summer days. This is leisurely biking that will be fun for kids, but may be too limited to interest adults.

Best Parking Lot: The state-beach parking lot.

Directions: Take Exit 62 from I-95 and head south along the 4-lane park entrance road for about 1.5 miles.

For More Information: The Bureau of Outdoor Recreation, Department of Environmental Protection, 165 Capital Avenue, Hartford, Connecticut 06106. Tel.: (203) 566-2304.

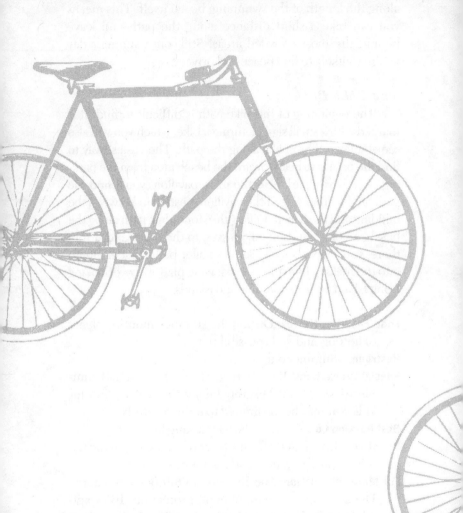

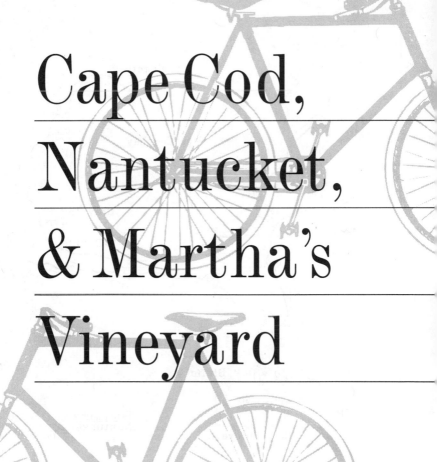

Cape Cod,

Nantucket,

& Martha's

Vineyard

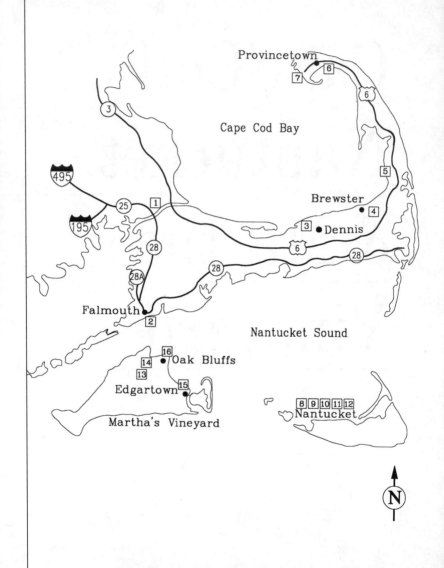

Cape Cod, Nantucket, & Martha's Vineyard

1. The Cape Cod Canal Recreation Area

BOURNE AND SANDWICH, MASSACHUSETTS

General Description:

Two 7-mile roads, wide and flat, running along both canal banks, closed to motorized traffic, with no road crossings.

Level of Difficulty: Very easy. A great place for young cyclists.

Type of Scenery: A "10" in entertainment value! A steady stream of boats, from tiny sailboats to mammoth tankers and Navy ships; 3 bridges to ride under, including the unique railroad bridge at Buzzards Bay; beaches and sea life; several excellent fishing spots.

Condition of Pavement: Excellent; much recent repaving.

General Background:

By the beginning of the twentieth century, Cape Cod had come to symbolize summertime and serenity to city folk. But to those who earned their living on the water, the phrase "Cape Cod" inspired terror. This long and crooked elbow of sandy land, poking far out into the Atlantic's Gulf Stream, is really just one huge sand dune, a remnant deposited by the receding glacier of the most recent Ice Age.

The glacier also left behind the extensive and shallow shoals that surround the Cape's outermost reaches. During the heyday of the American shipping era, the end of the nineteenth and beginning of the twentieth centuries, these dangerous shoals grounded at least a ship a week.

August Perry Belmont, one of the richest men in America, thought he saw a financial opportunity in this shipping crisis: Belmont dug the Cape Cod Canal, which opened 14 days before the Panama Canal, in July 1914. Belmont's canal, 100 feet wide and 15 feet deep, allowed only one ship at a time to pass and required constant dredging. Traffic lights at each end of the canal regulated the ships' flow.

Despite the problems, Belmont expected to make a profit: shipping companies would certainly prefer his route to the dangerous outer shoals. He was dead wrong. Even August Perry Belmont's capital couldn't fiance this ambitious venture.

After several serious accidents, Belmont began negotiating for a federal takeover. In 1928, the Army Corps of Engineers bought the canal for $11.5 million. The Corps widened and deepened the canal itself, and created along its banks a unique recreation area, visited by 4 million people a year by the 1990s.

The Bike Path:

The 2 paths of about 7 miles each are actually maintenance roads which have gradually come to be used by cyclists, walkers, joggers, and fishermen. Motorized traffic, except for the occasional Corps vehicle, is forbidden.

Since the service roads, quite wide and almost com-

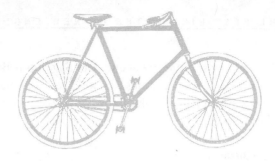

pletely flat, do not cross any roads, there's no better place to learn to ride a bike. Any vehicle *with* wheels but *without* a motor fits in. Our favorite sight: a young father, gliding on in-line skates, pushing along his 4-year-old son, who was regally enthroned on a tiny 2-wheeler.

Biking is only one of a huge variety of family activities available during the summer at this recreation area. At the Marine Traffic Control Center in Buzzards Bay, you can watch state-of-the-art computers monitor the canal's traffic. Along the canal banks are evening campfire programs and guided nature walks. Schedules of these activities are available from the Corps.

A Great Afternoon Excursion:

Swimming in the canal is forbidden; the current is too strong. But you can bike on the service road into Scusset State Beach Reservation, on the eastern end of the canal's mainland side. Drive into this beach and you pay a parking fee of about $5 (and also sometimes wait in line). Bike in and the beach is free. Park your car at the Sagamore Bridge canal-recreation-area parking lot (all canal lots are free), bike the 2.5 miles to Scusset Beach, put your bikes in the racks, enjoy the beach, then bike back.

If it's a busy summer weekend, the Sagamore Bridge lot may be full. Try the Herring Run lot. Many people stop at Herring Run just to look at the view; with patience, you'll find a spot.

Bike Path Distances:

The North Service Road (mainland side)

Total length:	7.2 miles
Railroad Bridge to Bourne Bridge:	1.3 miles
Bourne Bridge to Herring Run:	2.4 miles
Herring Run to Sagamore Bridge:	1.0 miles
Sagamore Bridge to Scusset Beach:	2.5 miles

The South Service Road (Cape side)

Total length:	6.8 miles
Western terminus to Railroad Bridge:	0.8 miles
Railroad Bridge to Bourne Bridge:	1.4 miles
Bourne Bridge to Sagamore Bridge:	2.4 miles
Sagamore Bridge to the Bulkhead:	2.2 miles

Special Precautions: (1) Bring a tire-patch kit! At low tides, gulls crack seashells on the service-road pavement. These broken shells slash tires as easily as broken glass.

(2) The canal can be a wind tunnel. On summer days, winds are often calm in the morning and build through the afternoon, frequently reaching gusts of 20 miles per hour later in the day. When you start out, note the wind's direction. It's often out of the southwest. Cycle into it; on your return trip, you'll pedal with rather than against the wind. Even strong cyclists tire unexpectedly in these velocities.

Food Facilities Nearby: Several sandwich shops at the Buzzards Bay end of the canal; clam shack across from the Herring Run rest area and parking lot; many restaurants near the Sandcatcher parking lot in Sandwich.

Restrooms: At each recreation area: Herring Run and Sagamore on the mainland side; Sandcatcher, Sandwich, Bourne, and Tidal Flats on the Cape side.

Best Parking Lot: The Sagamore Recreation Area and the Herring Run Recreation Area.

Directions: (1) From Route 3 from Boston, go almost all the way around the Sagamore Rotary, passing the Sagamore Bridge. Take the next right turn off the rotary. A sign says: "Canal." The parking lot is at the bottom of the road.

(2) From Routes 25 and 495, take the last exit before the bridge (Exit 2) to Buzzards Bay. Follow signs for Route 6 East, by going around the rotary and edging into the right-hand lane. Route 6 East goes under the Bourne Bridge and parallels the canal for several miles, although you won't be able to see the canal itself at first. After about 3 miles, on the right there will be a sign for the Herring Run parking lot, directly on your right. To get to the Sagamore Recreation Area parking lot, continue to the Sagamore Rotary and follow directions in (1) above.

For More Information: Engineer in Charge, U.S. Army Corps of Engineers, Cape Cod Canal Field Office, P.O. Box J, Buzzards Bay, Massachusetts 02532. Tel.: (508) 759-4431.

Recreation Hotline: (508) 759-5991 (for tides, fishing information, weather, and special programming).

2. The Shining Sea Bikeway

General Description:

A 3.1-mile bike path with short and gentle hills, running along the water's edge.

Level of Difficulty: Easy.

Type of Scenery: Saltwater coastline, swimming beach and saltwater ponds, Cape Cod houses with landscaped gardens.

Condition of Pavement: Excellent.

The Bike Path:

This little gem of a bike path, constructed on a railroad right-of-way, runs along Vineyard Sound from the town of Falmouth to the village of Woods Hole.

If you begin biking in Falmouth, you'll first cross a few streets and pass through a few backyards, but much of the path, even in town, has a countryside feel to it. This is because you're biking through wetland areas, where very little construction is allowed.

The middle stretch of path passes alongside several saltwater ponds, with a few resident mute-swan couples. Don't get too close. These birds are more dangerous than they look. There are several benches here where you can sit and look out over the ponds to the Vineyard Sound to the south.

Next, the path reaches the sea, and runs for more than

a mile along open oceanfront. You can stop for a few moments in the sun, for a rest or a picnic. Then the path climbs a very gradual hill, crosses a little wooden bridge, and ends at the Steamship Authority parking lot. Nearby, you can catch the ferry to Martha's Vineyard, and another set of bike paths.

Expect to find this popular path filled with strolling elderly couples and jogging mothers pushing baby carriages. In fact, the Shining Sea Bikeway is so well used that a Falmouth police officer patrols during the summer months on a bike.

This is not a bike path for people interested in speed. To *try* to avoid the crowds, go as early as possible. The parade doesn't really get moving along the Shining Sea until after noon.

Plans exist to extend the path from its current starting point to near the intersection of Palmer Avenue and Route 28. This will add about a mile to the path, avoiding the traffic congestion in town. The extension *may* be completed in the next few years.

A Great Day Excursion:

Park in Falmouth and pedal the 3.1 miles to Woods Hole. It will probably take you a half-hour or less. Woods Hole, a tiny town suffering from severe traffic congestion, encourages biking and has plenty of bike racks throughout the village.

Woods Hole, with its population of research scientists and working fishermen, has studiously avoided commercialism. Still, there are lots of interesting attractions: a drawbridge in the center of the village, large boats and ferries, a busy harbor with working fishing boats, and even a small aquarium, on Water Street, run by the Woods Hole Oceanographic Institution. There are several harbor boat rides, including one which dredges up sea life for the passengers to study. The village has good, inexpensive sandwich shops and ice-cream places, and ample picnic and grassy areas for families to sit down and rest.

Food Facilities Nearby: Inexpensive sandwich shops at Woods Hole end of bike path, within walking distance; in downtown Falmouth near other end.

Restrooms: In the Steamship Authority building in Woods Hole.

Special Precautions: None.

Best Parking Lot: The intersection of Woods Hole Road, Mill Road, and Route 28 (Locust Street). This parking lot is not well marked. At Woods Hole Road, opposite the parking lot, is a *very* small sign noting the start of the bikeway. If the parking lot looks full, go in anyway. Drive through this lot, almost to the back, and you'll find a second, nearly hidden parking lot.

Directions: From the Bourne Bridge, take Route 28 into Falmouth. After the road narrows from 4 to 2 lanes, you'll drive through a very commercial area. Signs will point toward Main Street on the left. Do not follow them, but bear slightly to the right, toward Woods Hole, and immediately begin looking for the dirt parking lot on the right.

For More Information: The town of Falmouth, 59 Town Hall Square, Falmouth, Massachusetts 02540. Tel.: (508) 548-7611.

3. The Cape Cod Rail Trail

General Description:

A mostly flat path of 25.8 miles, including 2 miles of on-street biking in the town of Orleans. Currently, New England's longest paved bike path.

Level of Difficulty: Easy for most of the trip. The easternmost segment, from Eastham to South Wellfleet, has some long but not-too-steep grades. The on-street ride, beside traffic, through Orleans includes some long but not steep inclines.

Type of Scenery: Cranberry bogs, saltwater ponds, and Cape scrub forests; freshwater swimming beaches; distant ocean vistas; industrial and commercial areas; several segments run alongside very busy roadways and highways; many road crossings.

Condition of Pavement: Poor near the western end; newly paved at the eastern end.

General Background:

When fashionable people began summering by the sea in the late 1800s, proper Bostonians became the first Cape Cod tourists. To accommodate them, the Old Colony Railroad Company laid tracks from Boston all the way to Provincetown, at the outermost tip. By 1873, Bostonians could escape the muggy city summer by taking the train to any number of seaside Cape villages—Sandwich, Hyannis, Orleans, Wellfleet, or Provincetown; the Boston-to-Provincetown journey required only 5 hours.

Automobile bridges opened over the Cape Cod Canal in 1935, dooming the trains. Passenger service east of Dennis ended in 1937; freight service anywhere on the Cape ended in the 1960s. Sand dunes and gnarly brambles buried the unused tracks. In a few places, paved automobile roads covered the railroad right-of-way.

In the late 1970s, the railroad bed reopened for travel. A state agency cleared out the overgrowth and paved the railroad bed, turning it into one of the nation's first rail trails. Cyclists and others could travel across bogs and through pine forests, just as their train-riding predecessors had a century earlier.

Spanning more than a third of the Cape's length, the

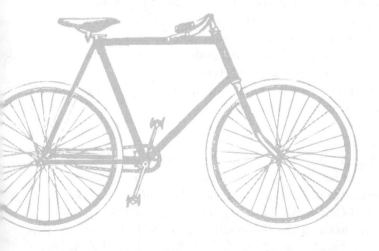

rail trail winds past freshwater kettle ponds where you can stop and swim, meanders through several protected ecosystems, passes over acres of saltwater tidal flats and freshwater marshes. Along the way you'll see a relatively pristine fishing village, some modern shopping areas where you can find some good lunch spots, and some great places to stop and picnic in the sun by the sea.

Several interesting spurs connect to the rail trail. In Brewster, an 8-mile paved trail branches off into the enormously popular Nickerson State Park. (See separate entry.) In Eastham, an on-road bike route of a bit less than a half-mile leads you to the National Seashore Visitor Center and onto the Nauset Trail, an esthetically exquisite bike path. (See separate entry.)

But: There are also some important drawbacks to consider when planning a ride here. This rail trail runs through some very developed areas, past industrial plants and through suburban housing developments. In several places the state was unable to acquire right-of-way separate from roadway; at times, the cyclist must either bike among cars on a busy street or along the shoulder of a busy highway. If you're riding with people who don't like traffic, these may be sections you choose to avoid.

The Bike Path:

The western end of the rail trail begins in Dennis; the eastern end, in South Wellfleet. The eastern half of the path is definitely prettier than the western half. Unless you plan to do the whole 25.8 miles, we suggest you begin in South Wellfleet. Although this segment of the path passes through industrial and backyard areas, the ride is a bit more rural. There are fewer road crossings, and you won't need to ride on any streets until you reach the town of Orleans.

The 6.2-mile leg from the South Wellfleet rail-trail parking lot to the turnoff for the Salt Pond Visitor Center of the Cape Cod National Seashore is the newest segment of the trail, officially opened in 1995. There are a few long, rather gradual grades in this segment which add interest but might be a bit strenuous for novice cyclists. The slight uphill climbs are more than compensated for by the beauty of the forest scenery. At several points along this segment, scenic spots overlook brooks and small ponds. A short segment winds through National Seashore wetlands and forests, an unspoiled area that's particularly pretty.

Some rail-trail and National Seashore brochures appear to imply that you can bike easily from the Cape Cod Rail Trail to the Visitor Center of the National Seashore in Eastham. Be wary of this, if you're with novices. The ride is about a half-mile, on-road, on winding streets with lots of cars during the summer season. To get to the Salt Pond Visitor Center from the rail trail, you must cross Route 6, the main east-west Cape highway. There is a traffic light to help you, but the highway is noisy and bustling. Currently, the turnoff from the rail trail onto Locust Road, the road you must take to get to the Visitor Center, is not marked along the rail trail itself; unless you're careful, you'll pass it by.

Continuing west along the rail trail itself, crossing Locust Road, you'll pass through bogs and marshes and ride past Boat Meadow River, noted in the writings of Henry David Thoreau (who, in fact, wrote a book about Cape Cod). This trail segment, from Locust Road to the on-road biking in Rock Harbor, is rather rural and enjoyable biking.

Next comes a segment of on-road biking, along Rock Harbor Road. If you don't mind traffic, you'll like this scenic area. But if you're worried about cars, these 2 miles might prove difficult. The Cape Cod Bay tidal flats extend for nearly a mile out into the water. You can leave your bike and walk at low tide, or even swim at high tide. Continuing through Orleans Center, you leave the built-up area again, passing through the saltwater marshes of Namskaket Creek, managed by the conservation commissions of the towns of Brewster and Orleans. The salt marsh flows into Cape Cod Bay, visible as a glistening blue band of salt water on the far horizon, just above the open marshland.

Next you'll arrive at Nickerson State Park, a distance of 7.9 miles from Locust Road in Eastham. Most maps show the bike paths of Nickerson State Park connecting with the rail trail. This is not quite accurate. To get to the park bike paths, you must turn into the park when you see the sign looming on the rail trail itself. Bike past the park restrooms and down the length of the parking lot. The park's bike path begins near the information office. (Nickerson State Park has the only public restroom facilities along the rail trail. There is also water available here.)

From Nickerson State Park west to Dennis, the rail trail runs through much more developed areas. You'll see more backyards; you'll have to cross more and more roads. Cars do not often stop for cyclists here, so exercise caution. There have been lots of accidents in this area.

Along Route 124 in Brewster, 3.6 miles west of Nickerson State Park, several kettle ponds provide opportunities for excellent freshwater swimming. The kettle ponds, gouged out during the last Ice Age, are deep and clean and spring-fed.

Farther on is the Pleasant Lake Store, a general store which has become so famous for its hospitality to rail-trail users that it is included in brochures published by the state's Department of Environmental Management.

Near the general store comes a *very* dangerous on-road section of the rail trail. Use caution. Cars speed on this highway. The rest of the ride is through heavily built-up areas, with many road crossings.

Bike Path Distances:

From Route 134 to Pleasant Lake Store, Harwich:	5.9
From Pleasant Lake Store to Route 124, Brewster:	2.1
From Route 124 to Route 137, Brewster:	0.9
From Route 137 to Underpass Road, Brewster	0.5
From Underpass Road to Millstone Road, Brewster:	1.5
From Millstone Road to Nickerson State Park, Brewster:	0.7
From Nickerson State Park to West Road, Orleans:	1.8
From West Road to Orleans Center:	0.8
From Orleans Center to Rock Harbor, Orleans:	1.1
From Rock Harbor to Courthouse, Orleans:	1.0
From Courthouse to Locust Road, Eastham:	2.7
From Locust Road to the Visitor Center:	0.5
From Locust Road to South Wellfleet Trail Head:	6.2

Special Hint:

The best time to bike on this, the longest of New England's paved paths, is definitely early spring or late fall.

November and December often have temperatures above 45 degrees—but no crowds. We were out on the path one Sunday afternoon in December and saw no other cyclists for most of the ride. Moreover, the roads on the Outer Cape are almost empty during these months, so the frequent road crossings are easier to negotiate.

Food Facilities Nearby: Some stores and sandwich shops along the roadside; a strip mall at the trail's start in Dennis; the Pleasant Lake Store in Harwich.

Restrooms: Nickerson State Park.

Special Precautions: Beware of dangerous road crossings and very heavy traffic on the path itself during peak hours.

    This path is a multi-use trail, open to equestrians as well as joggers, skaters, and walkers. There have been a few serious conflicts between cyclists and horseback riders. The best way to avoid accidents is to use caution when approaching horses, especially from behind. Warn riders ahead of time that you are coming.

Best Parking Lot: The South Wellfleet trail-head parking area; the Salt Pond Visitor Center of the Cape Cod National Seashore in Eastham; Nickerson State Park in Brewster; in Dennis, at the western beginning of the trail.

Directions: To the South Wellfleet trail head, take Route 6 until you just cross the South Wellfleet town line. Turn right onto LeCount Hollow Road. You will see the parking area immediately to your right.

    To get to the beginning of the trail in South Dennis, take Route 6 to Exit 9. Off the ramp, go south on

Route 134. Almost immediately, you will pass a strip mall and 2 traffic lights. On your left will be the dirt parking lot, with a sign. On busy days, it is very difficult to find parking here.

To get to the Nickerson State Park parking lot, take Exit 12 off Route 6. Head along Route 6A for 1.3 miles and look for park signs on the left.

To get to the Salt Pond Visitor Center, follow Route 6 to Eastham. The Visitor Center is along the highway and is very well marked. Then you must bike .5 mile along automobile roads—Salt Pond Road and Locust Road—to reach the rail trail. You might want to have young children walk their bikes, since drivers negotiate these curves at high speeds.

For More Information: Nickerson State Park, 3488 Main Street, Route 6A, Brewster, Massachusetts 02631-1521. Tel.: (508) 896-3491. (Send stamped, self-addressed envelope for return of information.)

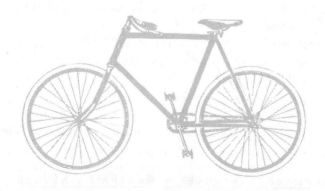

4. Nickerson State Park

General Description:

About 8 miles of bike paths, snaking through semi-developed parkland.

Level of Difficulty: Average to somewhat challenging.

Type of Scenery: Tall stands of red pine, oak, and scrub pine; a few ponds; near some well-traveled park roads and state camping areas.

Condition of Pavement: Quite rough in places.

General Background:

Nickerson State Park, 1,900 acres, has 420 camping sites, 4 huge freshwater ponds, and several smaller ones. These "kettle ponds" were formed 10,000 years ago, when the glaciers melted. Dependent on rainwater and groundwater rather than on streams, the ponds are deep and clear and clean. Their popularity for swimming and boating means this park is extremely busy throughout the summer. Getting a campsite here takes planning ahead, except during the late fall.

The Bike Path:

This path includes several loops that wind through wooded areas, but also parallel busy roads at times. The housing developments bordering the park are visible in a few spots. In several sections, the path follows power lines. These paths are fun to ride because of their roller-coaster climbs and twists, but you won't have the feeling of backwoods biking you get in Myles Standish State Forest. (See separate entry.)

The path begins at the park headquarters. This is also the only way to enter the park by automobile. (Some maps show other roads into the park, but they are gated and locked.) Park at the headquarters parking lot and look for the bike trail near the information office.

We divide these looped trails into an inner division and an outer division. The inner loop includes the Ober Trail and the Cedar Trail. If people in your party don't like hills, stick to this inner loop. There are a few long hills here, but most of the loop is somewhat flat—at least compared with the other park paths. The Ober Trail and Cedar Trail run through woodlands, often out of sight of roadways, and you'll still see some majestic stands of trees.

If, at the end of the Ober Trail, you get tempted by the sign pointing to Ruth Pond, as we did, be careful. Part of this trail descends quite steeply down a long hill. An unexpected switchback toward the bottom will be difficult to negotiate at high speeds.

Bike to Ruth Pond (there are several road crossings), where you can rest by the water. This pond, not a good swimming pond, is not accessible by automobile. We like the quiet respite from the midsummer noise.

Most maps show that the park's paths connect to the Cape Cod Rail Trail. This is not quite accurate. To find the rail trail, bike the length of the headquarters parking lot to the public restrooms. Beside the restrooms is a small semipaved pathway that leads to the rail trail. Nickerson State Park offers the only public restrooms for those who use the 25.8-mile rail trail.

Food Facilities Nearby: None, except a park store where a few things can be bought at high prices. Picnic tables are available.

Restrooms: Park headquarters; other areas throughout the park, during the summer months only.

Special Precautions: Be careful of long hills. Broken pavement in many places may make high speeds dangerous.

Best Parking Lot: Park headquarters.

Directions: Exit 12 off Route 6. Head west on Route 6A for 1.3 miles. Signs for park will be on your left.

For More Information: Nickerson State Park, 3488 Main Street, Route 6A, Brewster, Massachusetts 02631-1521. Tel.: (508) 896-3491.

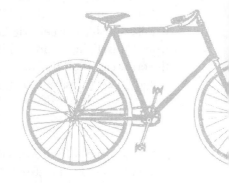

5. The Nauset Trail

General Description:

A 1.6-mile trail with many small, rolling hills, running from the Salt Pond Visitor Center, across Nauset Bay, down to Coast Guard Beach.

Level of Difficulty: Average.

Type of Scenery: Rare Cape hardwood forests, open marsh-lands with long wooden bridge, National Seashore swimming beach.

Condition of Pavement: Excellent.

General Background:

A century ago, when the shallow Cape Cod shoals wrecked a ship a week, vigilant men watched for trouble from Nauset's high, sandy cliffs. Seeing a floundering ship, the crew cast their tiny boats out into roiling sea. Officially called "The Lifesavers of Cape Cod," they were locally known as the "Guardians of the Ocean Graveyard." Their motto: "You have to go out, but you *don't* have to come back."

Below the cliffs, down a long flight of wooden stairs, is Cape Cod's most "must-see" beach—the beach that made Cape Cod famous, a beach with a view that steals the breath of the most jaded travelers. At low tide, breakers flow over the sandbars near the shore. Farther out to sea, almost to the horizon, breakers and whitecaps sparkle in the sunlight—evidence of the dangerous shoals just beneath the water's surface. The high sandy cliffs extend east into the distance. To the west lie wetlands, marsh, and miles of sand flats.

This beach is so popular in the summertime that an hour's wait for a parking spot is common. You'll also have to pay a parking fee of $5 to $10—unless you bike in on the Nauset Trail, after parking for free at the Salt Pond Visitor Center.

The Bike Path:

This bike path is esthetically exquisite! With its pretty curves, post-and-rail fencing, and gentle hills, this well-designed trail was clearly built to complement the area's natural beauty. The only other bike path in New England that achieves this level of design beauty is the Stowe Recreation Path in Vermont.

Pick up the trail at the far end of the Salt Pond Visitor Center; the beginning of the trail isn't obvious, but there is a small marker. The trail begins by winding through a grassy area bounded by rail fencing, then climbs slightly into stands of cedar and locust. Stands as extensive as these, once common, are now rare. Farther along, a high canopy shields the cyclist from the sun, making this path a good summertime alternative to the other National Seashore bike paths, which can be excessively hot.

After about a mile, these cool forests give way suddenly to the open lushness of Nauset Marsh. Across the wettest part of the marsh, the path leads over a long wooden bridge which sits below the high cliffs and white buildings of Coast Guard Beach. Pedaling through the marsh, over the bridge, and up the sand dunes, you'll feel as if you're biking back in time, pedaling through a peaceful world that disappeared decades ago.

When you get up to the top of the cliff, you'll return to the world of the automobile. If you're there in the summertime, there will, no doubt, be a long line of cars waiting for a place to park. You'll ride right past them and take advantage of the plentiful bike racks. You can stay for a short while, to look around from the clifftop viewing areas, or you can descend to the swimming beach and stay for the day.

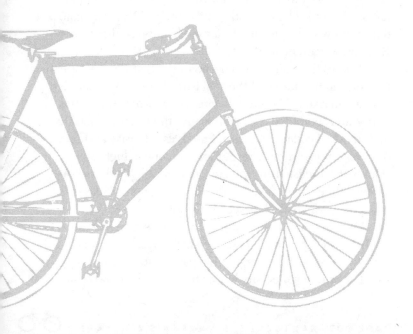

Special Note:

Some of the public-information brochures circulated by various agencies show that an extension of this bike path connects to the Cape Cod Rail Trail. This is not true. To reach the rail trail, you must cross Route 6 and bike for about a half-mile on busy streets. If you don't mind traffic, it's not a bad ride. If you're biking with novices, you might want to be cautious. For more information, see the Cape Cod Rail Trail entry.

Food Facilities Nearby: None. Bring picnic food.

Restrooms: Salt Pond Visitor Center, Coast Guard Beach.

Special Precautions: (1) The path is slightly hilly. Stay on the right side of the bike path, to avoid on-coming cyclists.

(2) In-line skating is forbidden on National Seashore paths.

Best Parking Lot: The Salt Pond Visitor Center of the Cape Cod National Seashore, Eastham. During the summer, when the beach parking costs from $5 to $10, the Visitor Center lot is free.

Directions: The Visitor Center is on Route 6 in Eastham.

For More Information: Cape Cod National Seashore Headquarters, South Wellfleet, Massachusetts 02663. Tel.: (508) 349-3785.

6. The Head of the Meadow Trail

THE CAPE COD NATIONAL SEASHORE

General Description:
A flat, 2-mile trail through scrub forests ending at a National Seashore swimming beach.

Level of Difficulty: Very easy.
Type of Scenery: Low bushes, open feeling; Pilgrim Spring, the first freshwater spring discovered by the Pilgrims.
Condition of Pavement: Poor. Lots of potholes and cracking.

General Background:
In November 1620, the Pilgrims saw their first land in the New World—the southern coast of Cape Cod. They sailed about a third of the Cape's length, but couldn't land because of the shallow shoals. Sailing back, they rounded the Cape's tip and entered the safer waters of what would become Provincetown, where they sheltered for several weeks before moving on to Plymouth.

The Pilgrims were desperate for fresh water. Unfortunately, then as now, this commodity was in short supply at the end of the sand spit that is Cape Cod. While they sheltered on the Cape's tip, they looked for water. Finally, after days of searching, they found a spring, now commemorated with a stone marker and a picnic table. You can stop in the middle of your bike ride and sit quietly in these peaceful surroundings, imagining the joyful relief of those thirsty travelers.

The Bike Path:

This almost completely flat path has much less scenic variety than the Nauset Trail but it has its own unique Outer Cape beauty. This is a harsh world, made up mostly of sand and the few hardy plants and scrubby trees that can make it through the windy winters.

The trees are stunted, and during the hot summer days there is no cooling overhead canopy here. The path winds around the base of several large sand dunes, eventually arriving at Head of the Meadow Beach. Though interesting, the path may not be fun for cyclists who want a bit of a challenge. We liked it because of the stop at Pilgrim Spring.

The path is *not* a good alternative entry to Head of the Meadow Beach. The bike-path parking lot on High Head Road, very small, is used by hikers and walkers, so you may have to wait for a parking space. Making matters worse, the lot has a 2-hour parking limit. You can bike over to Head of the Meadow Beach (it will only take you 10 minutes), but you can't stay long before it's time to return.

Food Facilities Nearby: None.

Restrooms: Port-o-potties and changing rooms at Head of the Meadow Beach. No running water.

Special Precautions: Very hot trail in the summertime, with no shade. Bring plenty of liquids.

Best Parking Lot: High Head Road. Very limited space. Get there early on summer days.

Directions: Off Route 6, just south of the Provincetown boundary.

For More Information: Cape Cod National Seashore Headquarters, South Wellfleet, Massachusetts 02663. Tel.: (508) 349-3785.

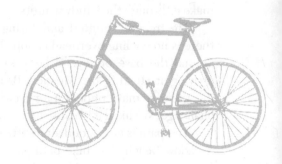

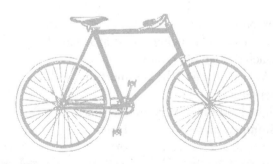

7. The Province Lands Trail

General Description:

Distinctive! A "must-do" ride! More than 7 miles of bike trails, a loop and 4 spurs, at the very tip of Cape Cod. You'll never see anything else quite like this bike path!

Level of Difficulty: Very challenging. Many long, steep grades and sharp turns. Hot! Hot! Hot!

Type of Scenery: Mesmerizingly wide-open vistas, high and open sand dunes reminiscent of Africa's Sahel, some covered with sparse scrub pine and dune grass; a beech-tree forest and isolated forest ponds; several swimming beaches.

Condition of Pavement: Generally good, but some cracking. Watch the sand: "walking dunes" can cover the path.

General Background:

The wind and waves erode the beaches farther to the west, along the Cape's southern coastline, and carry the grains of sand here, to the Province Lands. While the cliffs of Nauset Beach are slowly eroding, the tip of the Cape is actually *growing* 2 to 4 feet each year. Sand from Truro arrives in the Province Lands; the wind builds the huge dunes, grain by grain, until the size of these sand-mountains resembles those in the Sahara Desert.

The eerie spaciousness is exhilarating. No wonder the

air and light drew a colony of creative artists to this isolated world. If you're a strong enough cyclist to handle the hills and the heat, the trek is well worth it.

The Bike Path:

Don't push it here. Allow plenty of time for a leisurely trip. The 5.25-mile distance around the loop is deceiving. The long hills and sharp turns tire many cyclists, easily making this distance feel twice as long.

Anyway, you'll want time to look around. You'll want to stop and sit by the ponds, get off your bike at the crest of one of these huge dunes and look at the distant coastline, ride on some of the spurs to the saltwater beaches or hidden forests. It's an easy place to spend a day, out of the way of the Cape Cod summer crowds.

Despite its difficulty, this is a very popular trail. It's not really possible to get away from the crowds completely, but you'll avoid the worst by parking at the Beech Forest parking lot. The lot, which also has a picnic area, is U-shaped. Go all the way around the lot, park at the far tip of the U, and pick up the paved bike trail nearby. We suggest you start by heading *away* from Race Point Road, going into the forest. This way, the first third of your trip will be through cool forests, past the ponds, along bike paths that are somewhat hilly but not forbidding.

When you get out of the forest and hit the high and open dune, you can bike up and down one or two of them. If they're too daunting, you can turn back into the forests. You'll have seen some of the most spectacular views but won't be committed to long distances under the hot sun.

If you've followed the route suggested above and biked into the interior from the Beech Forest parking lot, about a quarter of the way along the loop you'll find your first spur, leading to Bennett Pond. Shortly after this, the forest thins and the hills begin. You'll go up and down several hills until you reach the open dunes.

To the left is the mile-long spur leading to Herring Cove Beach. With long roller-coaster-like sweeps up and down to the ocean, with higher and more frequent hills than anywhere else along the trail, this spur is the most difficult. The junction of the Herring Cove Beach spur and the main loop, marked by a sign, is a good halfway resting place. The intrepid cyclists in your party, who really want to do 2 extra miles in the sun, can pedal down and back. The others can wait and enjoy the scenery.

From the Herring Cove Beach spur, it's on to Race Point Beach. Here there is a long switchback descent, an underpass, and a long climb up the next dune. You can look into the distance and see the far-off cyclists coasting down the other dune, coming toward you.

Parking at the Race Point Beach lot is tight in the summer. Race Point Road, the road to this popular beach, is also the road to the municipal airport. The last leg of the bike path parallels Race Point Road. This is the least scenic section of the loop.

The segment from Race Point Beach to the Province Lands Visitor Center and the Beech Forest parking lot is similarly hilly. The cyclists in our party who were tired waited at Race Point Beach, while those with energy rode back to get the car.

Bike Path Distances:

Loop Trail:	5.25 miles
Herring Cove Beach spur:	1 mile
Race Point Beach spur:	.50 miles
Bennett Pond spur:	.25 miles
Race Point Road spur:	.25 miles

Food Facilities Nearby: None.

Restrooms: Herring Cove Beach, Race Point Beach, Province Lands Visitor Center, Beech Forest.

Special Precautions: (1) Sun, heat, hills! Wear a hat! Bring plenty of liquids.

(2) Be very careful of winds, which can be quite severe. If the winds seem strong, check park-service advisories.

(3) Definitely bring a park-service trail map with you. They are available from the wooden boxes at the trail heads. There are signs at the spurs in the loop path, but they are not easy to understand. Some have been defaced. We sat at several of these signs and watched group after group become confused.

(4) In-line skating is forbidden on National Seashore trails.

Best Parking Lot: Beech Forest picnic area.

Directions: Follow Route 6 almost all the way to the end of the Cape, to Provincetown. Turn right (north) on Race Point Road, and park almost immediately, at Beech Forest, on your left, marked by well-placed signs.

For More Information: Cape Cod National Seashore Headquarters, South Wellfleet, Massachusetts 02663. Tel.: (508) 349-3785.

8. The Milestone Road Bike Path

General Description:

A 6-mile flat path parallel to a busy road.

Level of Difficulty: Easy.

Type of Scenery: Heathland; open marshland; urban and suburban at the west end; quaint Siasconset Village at the east end.

Condition of Pavement: Good.

General Background:

Nantucket Island, one of the nation's oldest settlements, is surprisingly accessible by bike. The island, 14 miles long and 3 to 6 miles wide, hosts 5 bike paths ranging in length from 1.5 to 8.2 miles.

These paths, intended as major avenues of transportation on an island crowded with automobiles, are a great way to see this unique historic settlement. Islanders welcome tourists, but encourage them to leave their cars on the mainland.

The 5 bike paths span out like spokes in a wheel from the hub, Nantucket Town. Besides being the commercial center of the 50-square-mile island, this is where the ferry from the mainland docks, taking on and letting off vehicles several times a day. The tiny town, with its streets laid out in the 1720s, becomes quite crowded with traffic.

There are no bike paths in Nantucket Town. It is possible to find your way through the back streets and avoid some of the traffic, but many of these streets are cobblestone-covered and difficult to negotiate. We suggest, if you have children or novice cyclists in your party, that you plan on walking your bikes through the town.

The Bike Path:

The Milestone Road Bike Path parallels a busy road. Still, the heathland, scrub forests, and bogs make up a unique ecosystem that visitors find interesting. At the end of the bike path is a must-see village: Siasconset, famous for its small houses with their rose-covered trellises. Like the island's other settlements, Siasconset has a boom-and-bust history. In the seventeenth century, it was a fishing village. The men built one-room shacks to serve as temporary homes while they were fishing and shore-whaling at this end of the island. Eventually, some of the fishermen's wives wanted to come along on these expeditions. Kitchens and enclosed porches were added.

For decades, the fishing shacks lay empty. Then, during the 1880s, the fashionable set noticed Siasconset. Wealthy families built larger homes on the village outskirts; the New York theater-and-artist crowd bought the quaint little buildings for summer homes. A century later, the village is still a popular summer resort.

The Milestone Road Bike Path ends in Siasconset at the intersection of Main Street and New Street, at the west edge of town.

Food Facilities Nearby: Several small restaurants and sandwich shops in Siasconset, open during the summer months.

Restrooms: Most of the public beaches have restrooms open during season. Restrooms open to the public in Nantucket include those at the Steamship Authority and at the Visitor Information Center at the corner of Federal and East Chestnut Streets in Nantucket Town.

Special Precautions: Bring plenty of liquids for the ride. There are no stores or restaurants between Nantucket Town and Siasconset.

This path can become very crowded.

Best Parking Lot: None.

Directions: This path begins at the rotary east of Nantucket Town. The simplest way to get to the rotary from the ferry is to head up Main Street and turn left onto Orange Street. Orange Street enters the rotary. There is a bike-path sign on the right side of Milestone Road. Nantucket Town's Main Street is paved with cobblestones.

For More Information: The Nantucket Visitors Services Bureau, 25 Federal Street, Nantucket, Massachusetts 02554. Tel.: (508) 228-0925.

9. The Madaket Road Bike Path

General Description:

A 5.5-mile bike path, with lots of fun twists and turns, paralleling the automobile road from Nantucket Town to Madaket Beach.

Level of Difficulty: Average.

Type of Scenery: Heathland; wetlands and ponds; seaside village and seashore.

Condition of Pavement: Good.

General Background:

Madaket, one of the island's prettiest paths, ends at a very pleasant beach with bike racks but no public parking lot, making it a less-crowded shore area.

Two interesting historic sites lay near this path's start. At the intersection of Madaket and Quaker Roads is the Quaker cemetery. At one time, Quakers made up a major segment of the island's population. This cemetery contains many unmarked graves; until 150 years ago, the religion forbade headstones or grave markers. A half-mile beyond the cemetery are a boulder and plaque commemorating Abiah Folger Franklin, Benjamin Franklin's mother, born near that site in a house no longer standing.

The Bike Path:

If we had time to ride only one bike path on Nantucket, this would be it. Several marshes and saltwater ponds along the path have benches so cyclists and walkers can sit and enjoy the peaceful surroundings. There are some small hills to negotiate and some interesting woodlands. Although this path does parallel the road, it feels farther from the traffic than the Milestone Road path.

The path ends at the village of Madaket, with its cluster of modern beach homes, where you bike on a somewhat widened sidewalk. At Madaket Beach, you can park your bike and walk along the beach. With no public parking lot, the beach is less crowded, although there is a well-used 4-wheel-drive beach-access road.

Food Facilities Nearby: None. Bring plenty of liquids. You'll be biking in the sun most of the way over rolling hills.

Restrooms: Madaket Beach, during the summer months.

Special Precautions: This path is sometimes quite windy. If you plan to bike to Madaket Beach and back, the strong winds can make the 11-mile round trip feel like 22 miles.

Best Parking Lot: None.

Directions: The simplest way to get to this bike path is to take Main Street out of town all the way to the Soldiers' and Sailors' Monument. Main Street, a cobblestone street, forks to the right; take that right. Very soon you will see another fork in the road. The left fork will be Madaket Road. The Madaket Road Bike Path begins in a few blocks.

For More Information: The Nantucket Visitors Services Bureau, 25 Federal Street, Nantucket, Massachusetts 02554. Tel.: (508) 228-0925.

10. The Cliff Road Bike Path

NANTUCKET ISLAND, MASSACHUSETTS

General Description:

A 1.5-mile bike path, paralleling Cliff Road, connecting to the Madaket Road Bike Path.

Level of Difficulty: Average, some hills.
Type of Scenery: The early settlement area of Nantucket; historic homes, gardens, and village scenery.
Condition of Pavement: Good.

General Background:

When you ride through this historic neighborhood, you'll be riding through our nation's earliest history. The first European settlement on the island was built here, around 1660. Called Sherburne, the settlement was abandoned in the 1720s, when the Europeans moved to Nantucket Town, favoring the new site because of its superior harbor. None of the original buildings remain.

Indians, of course, had lived on the island for centuries, drawn here because the isolation protected them from predators and other tribes.

The Bike Path:

This short side path intersects the Madaket Road path at about one-third the length of Madaket. For a short ride, try biking out of Nantucket Town on the Cliff Road path and returning to town on the Madaket Road path. For a longer ride, you can take Cliff Road out to the Madaket path and ride to Madaket Beach.

Food Facilities Nearby: None.

Restrooms: Madaket Beach, during the summer months; restrooms in Nantucket Town.

Special Precautions: Watch out for traffic.

Best Parking Lot: None.

Directions: To get to the Cliff Road Bike Path, you must bike on Cliff Road itself for a distance. If you don't mind the traffic, the road is worth seeing. This may not be the best place to take young children, unless everyone is willing to walk bikes. To get to Cliff Road, turn right on South Beach Street near Steamboat Wharf. Turn left on Easton, and right onto Cliff Road.

For More Information: The Nantucket Visitors Services Bureau, 25 Federal Street, Nantucket, Massachusetts 02554. Tel.: (508) 228-0925.

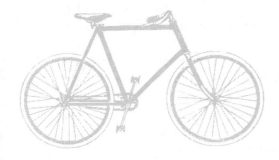

11. The Surfside Road Bike Path

NANTUCKET ISLAND, MASSACHUSETTS

General Description:

A 2.2-mile, flat path leading to a terrific beach, paralleling busy Surfside Road.

Level of Difficulty: Very easy.

Type of Scenery: Suburban construction, lots of homes and traffic; great walking beach!

Condition of Pavement: Good.

The Bike Path:

This is definitely a "get-you-there" path, designed for functionality rather than beauty. But it does the job, getting you from town to this terrific, scenic beach, a place where you can lock your bike and walk along the water for hours at a time.

Surfside Beach is a very popular summer beach. Expect crowds at the beach and on the path as well, if you decide to go during peak hours. Most of the ride will be through suburban neighborhoods, until you arrive at the beach itself. Although there are hundreds of bike racks, they will be full on a summer weekend.

Food Facilities Nearby: During the summer months, a hot-dog-and-ice-cream stand at Surfside Beach; some shops and stores at the beginning of the path.

Restrooms: During the summer months, at Surfside Beach.

Special Precautions: Watch for traffic.

Locally, this spot has a reputation for bike theft. Bring a heavy-duty bike lock.

Best Parking Lot: The Surfside Beach lot is very small and usually full in season. The point of the bike path is to help visitors and islanders alike avoid the drive from town. Leave your car in town; take your bike.

Directions: The simplest route is to take Main Street out of town, turn left onto Pleasant Street, then right onto Atlantic Avenue to Surfside Road. Main Street is a cobblestone street.

For More Information: The Nantucket Visitors Services Bureau, 25 Federal Street, Nantucket, Massachusetts 02554. Tel.: (508) 228-0925.

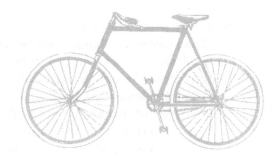

12. The Polpis Road Bike Path

General Description:

An 8.2-mile path ending in Siasconset near the Mile-stone Road Bike Path, allowing you to make a loop around the eastern end of Nantucket Island with only a short on-street ride.

Level of Difficulty: Average.

Type of Scenery: Heathland, wetlands, marsh, and cranberry bogs; some large homes and resort areas; the village of Siasconset.

Condition of Pavement: New.

General Background:

This long-time-coming, much-looked-forward-to path required more than $3 million to build, 119 easements from private landowners, and a decade of planning.

The 119 easements were all granted voluntarily, a real achievement that stems from the islanders' support of bike paths as an alternative to road construction. Nevertheless, construction of this path, once expected to be completed by 1989, required considerable dedication and patience. Most islanders feel the wait has been worthwhile.

The Bike Path:

"Polpis" is a Native American word meaning "the

divided or branched harbor." There is indeed such a harbor, about 6 miles east of Nantucket Town. From the seventeenth century until the early twentieth century, this most successful farming community had peat bogs, salt factories, and even mills where sheep's wool was processed into cloth.

This winding bike path begins at the rotary, also the beginning of the Milestone Road Bike Path. The Nantucket Life Saving Museum is about halfway down the Polpis Road path. Just a bit farther, on the right, is a cranberry bog, the Windswept Cranberry Bog, privately owned but open to the public for strolling. (They prefer that you not ride bikes over the bog dikes.) As you continue east along the path, you come to a golf course and Wauwinet Road, which leads to a wildlife sanctuary and a private residential community. In the distance, on the bluff near Siasconset, is the Sankaty Light, visible 29 miles out to sea. This lighthouse, nearly 150 years old, is likely to be destroyed by the sea; natural beach erosion is gradually wearing away its foundation.

The path ends in Siasconet, the village of rose-covered cottages, where you can pick up the Milestone Road Bike Path back to Nantucket Town. Since the Polpis Road has hills and the Milestone Road is relatively flat, we suggest you ride out to Siasconset on the Polpis Road and back to Nantucket Town on the much easier Milestone Road.

Food Facilities Nearby: None along the path; sandwich shops and restaurants in Siasconset, during the summer months.

Restrooms: None as yet; may be built.

Special Precautions: This path skirts the hilly northern coast of the island and can be quite windy. Be prepared for headwinds. Be in condition for this ride. Bring liquids.

Best Parking Lot: None.

Directions: This path begins at the rotary east of Nantucket Town. The simplest way to get there from the ferry is to head up Main Street and then turn left onto Orange Street, a street with very heavy traffic. Orange Street enters the rotary. You can see the signs for Polpis Road from the rotary.

For More Information: The Nantucket Visitors Services Bureau, 25 Federal Street, Nantucket, Massachusetts 02554. Tel.: (508) 228-0925.

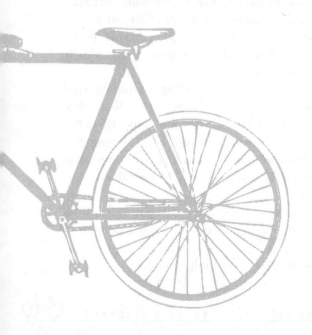

13. The Manuel F. Correllus State Forest Bike Paths

MARTHA'S VINEYARD, MASSACHUSETTS

General Description:

A mostly flat, loop path that runs along the circumference of this state forest, adding up to 12.8 miles of paths, including its several spurs.

Level of Difficulty: Easy.

Type of Scenery: Scrub pine and oak; open fields; some farmland; a few small housing developments.

Condition of Pavement: Good in some places, excellent in others.

General Background:

This forest of about 4,300 acres is a great refuge if you want to escape the beach frenzy. When the coastal bike paths are summer mob scenes, these forest paths are often nearly empty. Most of this woodland is located on fairly flat land. The scenery is sometimes monotonous, but we found the forest a place of peace in the midst of mayhem.

This state forest began, in fact, as a refuge for the last surviving Martha's Vineyard heath hens. The hope was that the birds would like the isolated forest enough to begin breeding again and replenish the disappearing species. This, unfortunately, did not come to pass. The heath hens disappeared from the earth, but the forest remains.

The Bike Path:

Throughout the forest is a latticework of wide, flat dirt-and-sand roads, used by horses, joggers, hikers, and cyclists. They are forbidden to motorized vehicles.

The paved paths are meant specifically for biking, although other activities are permitted. These paths run mostly around the perimeter of the forest, sometimes nearing automobile roads, but not too often. These are great paths for families and beginning cyclists, because of their easy grades and lack of crowds. There are a few more difficult hills along the path at the eastern end, but even these are suitable for beginning riders.

To ride a complete loop, begin at the parking lot on Barnes Road, head west along the perimeter, then south to West Tisbury Road. You'll travel south of the Martha's Vineyard Airport (yes, they've put an airport in the middle of this forest, but it's less annoying than you might think), then turn left again at Barnes Road, heading back toward Vineyard Haven and Oak Bluffs. You should see signs pointing to these towns.

Rather than turning left onto Barnes Road, you can continue along West Tisbury Road to go to Edgartown. This bike path, however, currently extends past Barnes Road toward Edgartown for only a short distance. The rest of the way, you'll have to bike on the busy road.

If you don't mind on-road riding, you can pick up the Beach Road bike path in Edgartown, at the bottom of West Tisbury Road and bike back to Oak Bluffs, where you can take your life in your hands by biking back along the busy automobile road to Vineyard Haven, or you can find a taxi with a bike rack.

Food Facilities Nearby: None near the state forest. Bring something to drink.

Restrooms: In airport, in Edgartown, at the visitor center on Church Street, just off Main Street; in Oak Bluffs, next to the Steamship Authority terminal, Seaview Avenue, also on Kennebec Avenue; also on the harbor next to Our Market; in Vineyard Haven, near the Steamship Authority dock, off Water Street.

Special Precautions: To get to this state forest, you'll either have to take a taxi or bike along very heavily traveled automobile roads.

Best Parking Lot: There are several parking lots surrounding the state forest. We like the small Barnes Road lot, but you shouldn't have trouble on most days finding a parking space if you do drive to the forest.

Directions: From the Edgartown–Vineyard Haven Road Bike Path (see next entry), heading toward Edgartown, turn right onto Barnes Road. If you're biking, this segment does not yet have a separated bike path. It's a short distance. You'll see several small parking areas and some open roads heading into woodlands on your right. If you look here, you'll see a paved bike path beside the dirt road.

For More Information: Martha's Vineyard Chamber of Commerce, P.O. Box 1698, Beach Road, Vineyard Haven, Massachusetts 02568. Tel.: (508) 693-0085.

14. The Edgartown– Vineyard Haven Bike Path

MARTHA'S VINEYARD, MASSACHUSETTS

General Description:
A 6.5-mile hilly path closely paralleling a busy highway.

Level of Difficulty: Average.
Type of Scenery: Suburban homes; some countryside.
Condition of Pavement: Good.

General Background:
The latest glacier to pass through this area created the odd division between up-island and down-island geology. The southeastern side of the island is an outwash plain; its flatness was created from the glacier's meltwater. A geological cousin to the Great Plains, the Martha's Vineyard outwash even contains plants and animals similar to those of the Great Plains.

The remainder of the island is a bit more rugged, as you'll realize if you bike this path. There are rolling hills here, with wide basins and inclines that are longer than you might expect in this area, although they are not extremely steep.

The Bike Path:

This is a utilitarian bike path meant to get cyclists safely from town to town, reducing the need for cars. The path can be physically challenging to beginning cyclists and doesn't offer much in the way of scenic beauty.

It does have two major attributes: (1) It will get you to Edgartown with a minimal amount of on-road biking. (2) It will take you to some really enjoyable bike paths running through the state forest in the island's center. (See preceding entry.) Be aware that the Edgartown–Vineyard Haven Road Bike Path does not yet connect directly with the state-forest bike-path system. There are plans to complete this short link, but no date has been set for the work.

Food Facilities Nearby: Vineyard Haven has lots of good sandwich shops and informal restaurants. This is a dry

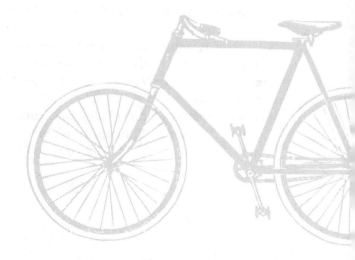

town. You cannot buy any alcohol in stores or restaurants. Most restaurants allow patrons to bring their own.

Restrooms: In Edgartown, at the visitor center on Church Street, just off Main Street; in Oak Bluffs, next to the Steamship Authority terminal, Seaview Avenue; also on Kennebec Avenue; also on the harbor next to Our Market; in Vineyard Haven, near the Steamship Authority dock, off Water Street.

Special Precautions: To get to and from this path, you'll have to use busy streets.

Best Parking Lot: None. See Beach Road entry.

Directions: To get to State Road from the ferry: follow boat traffic onto Water Street (a left turn). At "Five Corners" Intersection, make right turn and go up the hill. Continue until the intersection with Edgartown Road and make a left onto it.

This is your road. For a very short distance, you must bike on the road itself. But the wide parking/biking lane soon gives way to an actual bike path, completely separated from the road.

For More Information: Martha's Vineyard Chamber of Commerce, P.O. Box 1698, Beach Road, Vineyard Haven, Massachusetts 02568. Tel.: (508) 693-0085.

15. The Katama Road Bike Path

General Description:

A 2.6-mile, flat path to a very popular public beach, paralleling a busy road.

Level of Difficulty: Easy.
Type of Scenery: Upscale real estate; dairy farms; open space; beach.
Condition of Pavement: Good.

General Background:

Bartholomew Gosnold, a stray English sea captain who was actually looking for Virginia, came across this island accidentally in the first decade of the seventeenth century.

Even though there were already people living there — the Wampanoags—Gosnold decided he had "discovered" the island, and elected to name it after his daughter. Some of his passengers, having lost patience with a captain who couldn't find his real destination, elected to leave the ship and make their home on this land, rather than continue looking for Virginia.

These few founded Edgartown, the island's first European settlement, named after the son of the Duke of York. Edgartown, an important seaport for several centuries, has a rich maritime history. In the tiny town center are the Old Whaling Church, the Vineyard Museum, the Vincent House Museum, and the Dr. Daniel Fisher House, all worth visiting. Nearby is Chappaquiddick Island, a quite beautiful island where you'll find some pleasant on-road biking.

The Bike Path:

This fairly flat path leads from the town to the public beach, letting you glimpse a bit of the island's expensive real estate. On one side of the bike path you'll see homes of some of Edgartown's wealthy families. On the other side of the path, against all odds, cows and dairy farms not only survive but thrive. If you're seeking water views, you'll get them at the end of the path, at the public beach.

Food Facilities Nearby: In Edgartown.

Restrooms: In Edgartown, at the visitor center on Church Street, just off Main Street; in Oak Bluffs, next to the Steamship Authority terminal, Seaview Avenue on Kennebec Avenue; on the harbor next to Our Market; in Vineyard Haven, near the Steamship Authority dock, off Water Street.

Special Precautions: None.

Best Parking Lot: None. See special entry under the Beach Road Bike Path.

Directions: This path begins at the joining of South Water Street, Clevelandtown Road, and Katama Road. If you're biking from the Edgartown ferry, take Water

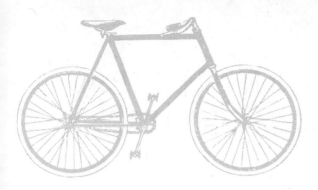

Street southwest out of Edgartown, and you'll soon come to the bike path on your left.

If you're biking from the Beach Road Bike Path, you must bike on the street for a short distance to connect up with this bike path. Continue along Upper Main Street to Cooke Street, then turn right onto Pease's Point Way, and bend to the left, to Katama Road.

For More Information: Martha's Vineyard Chamber of Commerce, P.O. Box 1698, Beach Road, Vineyard Haven, Massachusetts 02568. Tel.: (508) 693-0085.

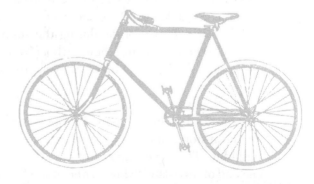

16. The Beach Road Bike Path

General Description:

A 4.4-mile, fairly flat path that runs along the ocean's edge, closely paralleling one of the island's busiest summertime roads.

Level of Difficulty: Easy.
Type of Scenery: Ocean beach and saltwater pond.
Condition of Pavement: Some cracking.

General Background:

Only 7 miles from Cape Cod, Martha's Vineyard is as different from Nantucket as nouveau is from antique. The 100-square-mile Martha's Vineyard, twice the size of Nantucket, is about 23 miles long and 9 miles wide. The winter population of 12,000 peaks during the summer at more than 100,000. Less than an hour by boat from Woods Hole on Cape Cod, Martha's Vineyard is very accessible to day-trippers.

If Nantucket is somewhat monochromatic, Martha's Vineyard thrives on diversity. People come to Nantucket for the history; they come to Martha's Vineyard for the social life. The richest and most famous own property on one end of this island, while on the other, hordes of college students summer in inexpensive rooming houses. Even if world leaders vacation here (Bill Clinton vacationed here, dining with Bill Styron), the island is anything but exclusive. You can bring your bike for the day and visit for the cost of a ferry ticket, or you can stay overnight in very inexpensive boarding houses, or vacation in old-fashioned hotels at a cost of hundreds of dollars a night. (From June through Columbus Day Weekend, you'll do best with advance reservations.)

The Bike Path:

The Beach Road Bike Path, the island's most scenic path, has some terrific saltwater views. Unfortunately, it also runs beside a busy beach highway. Still, if you don't mind the noise and fumes, this path is a great ride.

For much of its length, the path is bordered on one side by ocean and on the other by the saltwater Sengekontacket Pond, part of the Felix Neck Sanctuary, a wildlife sanctuary maintained by the Audubon Society.

If you're staying overnight, try biking along this path in the early-morning hours, before the sun-'n'-fun crowd gets up. In the early-morning peacefulness, you'll see nesting osprey, terns, and piping plovers. At the right time of year and at an early hour, you might be able to watch the osprey cruising low over the water, bringing up fish. Take binoculars. This area is one of the most popular in New England for serious bird-watching.

Strung out along much of the path's length are public swimming areas, in both the saltwater pond and the ocean. There is also good fishing and shellfishing, but you must have a license.

If you're coming over on the ferry for a day-trip and

want to do only one bike path, we suggest this one. The best way to get to the path from the ferry is to select a boat that docks in Oak Bluffs (during the summer months you can choose from several different ferry destinations), bike along the Beach Road path to Edgartown, spend several hours in this historic village, then bike back in the early evening to catch the ferry to the mainland.

Food Facilities Nearby: Many restaurants and sandwich shops in both towns.

Restrooms: In Edgartown, at the visitor center on Church Street, just off Main Street; in Oak Bluffs, next to the Steamship Authority terminal, Seaview Avenue; also on Kennebec Avenue.

Special Precautions: Winds from the ocean sometimes provide a cooling breeze, but easily develop into formidable headwinds. During the summer, the windiest time is often late afternoon, right before sundown.

If you plan to stop and swim or walk around, bring a bike lock. Bike theft is increasing. There are few bike racks along this path.

Best Parking Lot: None. Don't bring a car to the island if you don't have to. The taxi system and shuttle-bus system is extensive; some public-transportation vehicles have bike racks.

A Special Note on Transportation: During some winter and spring months, public ferries do not run to Oak Bluffs or Edgartown. You must come and go from the island by way of Vineyard Haven, the island's tourist and commercial center. You can bike from Vineyard Haven to Oak Bluffs, about 3 miles along the automobile road, but the road is narrow and busy, even during the off-season.

If you want to get to the Beach Road path and see Edgartown, you might arrange ahead of time to be met at the ferry by a shuttle or taxi with a bike rack. They'll also pick you up and take you back to the ferry by arrangement. For the most precise information, call the island's Chamber of Commerce.

Directions: To get to this path, you must bike on roads for about a half-mile from the Oak Bluffs ferry. Get off the ferry and look for signs to Seaview Avenue. This becomes Beach Road at the edge of town, which is where the bike path begins. Consider walking your bike till you reach the path; traffic is heavy.

For More Information: Martha's Vineyard Chamber of Commerce, P.O. Box 1698, Beach Road, Vineyard Haven, Massachusetts 02568. Tel.: (508) 693-0085.

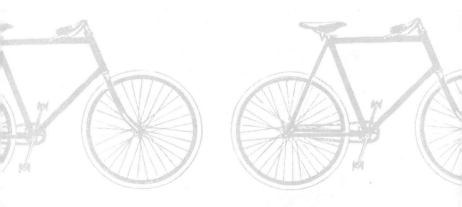

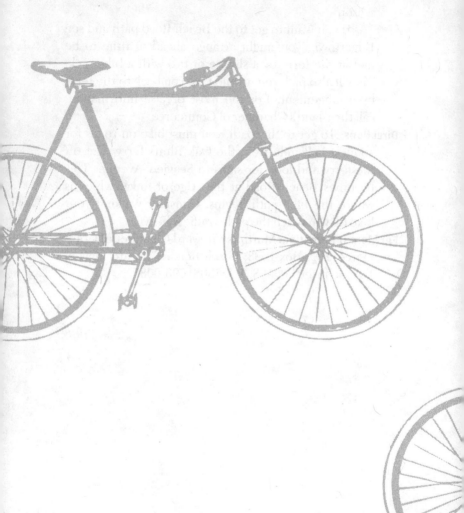

Mainland
Massachusetts

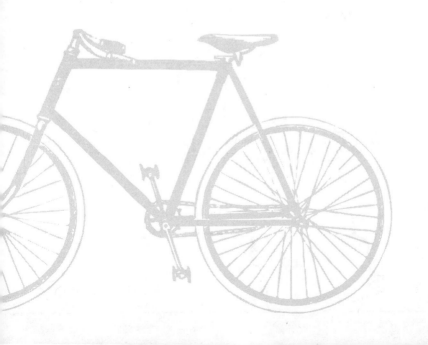

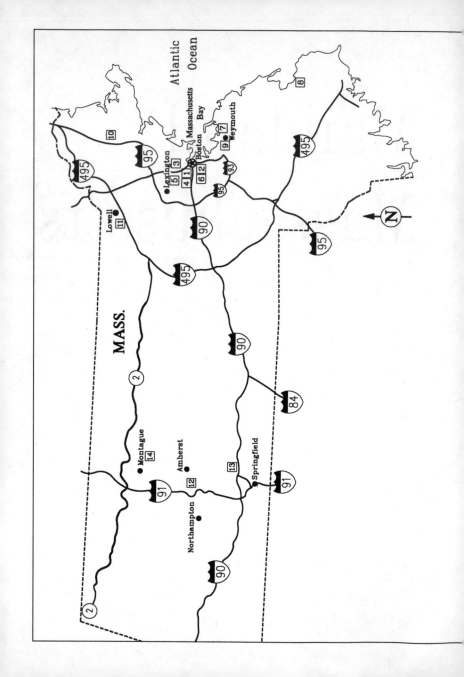

Massachusetts

1. The Dr. Paul Dudley White Bike Path

General Description:

A 17.7-mile loop along both banks of the Charles River, from Boston's Museum of Science, at the mouth of the river, to the Watertown Bridge, about 9 miles upriver.

Level of Difficulty: Easy.

Type of Scenery: The finest of Boston cityscape; the Charles River Esplanade; the campus buildings of MIT, Harvard, Boston University; sailboats near the mouth of the river, crew boats farther upstream.

Condition of Pavement: Good in some sections; very poor in some sections, bordering on dangerous at a few spots.

General Background:

Paul Dudley White was Dwight Eisenhower's personal physician, the man who first publicly emphasized the connection between regular exercise and healthy hearts. As a fitting honor to White's efforts, this path around the Charles River was built nearly 30 years ago. Although it has been neglected since then (there are several very dangerous spots), it's still a great way to see the Boston metropolis, especially if you're visiting for the first time.

Along the ride you'll have the Charles River on one side, while on the other you'll have the city itself: Boston's famous universities, including Harvard and MIT; the Charles River Esplanade, with its beautifully designed footbridges, where the Boston Pops summer orchestral performances are held; views of Beacon Hill, topped by the golden dome of the State House; the modern buildings of East Cambridge, the lair of the wealthy high-tech companies.

Even if you've been around Boston a while, cycling along the Dr. Paul Dudley White Bike Path is likely to give you a different perspective from any you'll get in an automobile.

The Bike Path:

If you begin cycling from the Nonantum parking lot in Newton, head downstream toward the mouth of the Charles River. You'll bike through a narrow strip of parkland sandwiched in between the road and the river. This strip widens after several miles, so you'll feel a bit more separated from the traffic.

At this point, you begin cycling through the collegiate area. If it's a warm spring day, count on the presence of lots of students from the nearby universities. At about the middle of the 9-mile stretch from Watertown to the Museum of Science, you'll see the buildings of Harvard University across the river. There are several bridges here on which cyclists can safely cross the river, in case you want to bike only half the 17.7-mile-loop path.

If you continue, you'll see the Charles widen into an open and wind-whipped body of water. Instead of canoes and rowing shells, you'll see flocks of sailboats. You'll come to the Esplanade, some of the most pleasant city biking you'll find anywhere in the world. Esplanade planners have separated the bike and walking paths, so you shouldn't have to navigate around strolling tourists. You'll pass mounted police on their huge, quiet horses; playgrounds filled with kids; lawns filled with lounging students; tennis courts and park benches. From time to time, you'll catch the wafting aroma of a nearby restaurant, and then the smell of the salt air as you near the mouth of the river.

At the mouth of the river is the Museum of Science, actually built over the water. You cross to the other bank of the river on the far side of the museum, by way of a widened sidewalk.

You'll have to look around a bit to find your way; as on most bike paths inside Route 128, signage along the Paul Dudley White is minimal. Before you get to the Museum of Science, the path seems to lead to a police-station parking lot. Go through that parking lot. You'll find yourself in front of the museum. On the other bank of the river, the path resumes.

As you bike down the East Cambridge side of the Charles, across the river you'll see an almost perfect, unobstructed view of Beacon Hill, with its historic town houses and its gold-domed State House. From this perspective, Beacon Hill looks like a busy little anthill.

Continuing in the direction of Harvard, crossing the Longfellow Bridge, you begin to bike along Memorial Drive; here the bike path and the automobile highway are divided only by very low cement curbing. This is a dangerous spot, since the path hugs the busy highway too closely.

A fall here would throw the cyclist into the path of oncoming traffic.

Eventually, the land beside the river widens out into parkland again. By the time you reach the Harvard University area, there is a strip of grassland between the path and the road. Past Harvard the strip widens even more. Eventually, the path is bordered by wide lawns and runs at some distance from the highway.

From Harvard to the Watertown Bridge, much of the path runs through scenic sections that are often quite close to the riverbank and well separated from the road traffic and noise. At times, however, you will be biking near traffic. At Watertown Square, because of the confusing traffic situation, you may want to walk your bike over the Watertown Bridge. The bike path over the bridge is not much more than a sidewalk. Across the bridge, the path picks up again as separate pavement, running through a narrow strip of parkland along the riverbank.

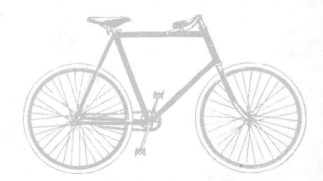

A Great Day Excursion:

If you want to ride the Dr. Paul Dudley White Bike Path all the way around (it's a terrific thing to do at least once in your life), but don't want to do 17.7 miles at once, consider breaking up the ride by visiting the Museum of Science for several hours. If you begin hiking at Watertown Square or at the Nonantum parking lot, you'll come to the museum at about the halfway point of your ride. Hitch up your bike at the bike rack, look around the museum, then mount up and ride back. Unless there's a strong wind or a large crowd (likely on a warm spring day), neither leg of this easy ride should take much more than an hour.

Food Facilities Nearby: Surprisingly, not many conveniently nearby. Bring your own drinks and picnic food.

There is a small restaurant in the Museum of Science.

Restrooms: None.

Special Precautions: There are several very dangerous street crossings, which you must navigate without the benefit of crossing lights.

Long sections of this path run next to major traffic arteries—Storrow Drive and Memorial Drive. There is no protective barrier, other than a small cement curb, between the path and the highway.

Count on crowds in the college areas on warm afternoons.

Best Parking Lot: There are many, many parking areas along this bike path, on both sides of the Charles River. You won't have any trouble finding a parking space.

We like the parking areas closer to the Watertown Bridge, which don't require negotiating the downtown Boston traffic. You can park east of the Watertown Bridge in Watertown, along the road itself, but we prefer the Daly Memorial Ice Skating Rink parking lot on Nonantum Road, which runs along the Newton side of the Charles River.

Directions: To get to Watertown Bridge from the Massachusetts Turnpike, take Exit 17. To get to the Watertown side of the river, follow signs for Galen Street and for Watertown. You will come to a large and complicated intersection; this is Watertown Bridge and Watertown Square. After Watertown Bridge, veer sharply to the right; you can park here and bike, or you can drive along this road to several municipal parking lots.

To get to the parking lot of the Daly Memorial Ice Skating Rink (our favorite parking area), along the Newton side of the Charles River, take Exit 17 from the Massachusetts Turnpike. Follow the signs for CharlesBank and Nonantum Roads. Nonantum Road parallels the Charles River. The ice skating rink parking lot is less than a mile east of the Watertown Bridge.

For More Information: The Metropolitan District Commission, 1400 Soldiers Field Road, Brighton, Massachusetts 02135. Tel.: (617) 727-4708.

2. The Stony Brook Reservation Bike Path

General Description:

A 3.7-mile path, much of it a large loop that twists around, climbing the steep granite hills of this urban forest.

Level of Difficulty: Challenging.
Type of Scenery: Woodlands; small ponds; large rock outcroppings.
Condition of Pavement: Poor

General Background:

The Metropolitan District Commission (MDC), whose park system ranges over 43 municipalities around Boston, was formed in 1893 to administer the region's park system. The commission quickly acquired the 475 acres of the Stony Brook Reservation, an elongated park that snakes around in an odd shape through West Roxbury and Hyde Park, southwest of Boston.

At the park's center is Turtle Pond, a small freshwater pond where people catch sunfish and perch. Stony Brook runs from Turtle Pond to the southern section of the reservation, where you'll find playing fields, tennis courts, an ice-skating rink, a pool, and picnic areas.

The Bike Path:

This winding woodland bike path is lots of fun, with surprises and challenges at every bend. Unfortunately, this wonderful facility is also the worst-maintained bike path we've ever seen. Large chunks of pavement, some 2 or 3 feet in diameter, have been eroded, creating potholes that are deep and quite dangerous.

It's almost impossible to find this ride. Don't bother to look for signs; there aren't any. Nor are there parking facilities to speak of. Visitors often park on the sides of the busy parkway that runs through the reservation.

Food Facilities Nearby: None.

Restrooms: None.

Special Precautions: The MDC doesn't patrol this park well. It's not a good area to visit after dark. Lock your vehicles.

Best Parking Lot: There really isn't one. Cyclists park along the road.

Directions: From Route 128, take Route 1 North for 1.2 miles. Turn right onto Washington Street and drive for 2 miles. Turn right onto LaGrange. At the bottom of the hill is the parkway that runs through the reservation. Turn right and look for the paved bike path that runs through the woods. There is no special parking lot for the path, so you'll have to depend on roadside parking.

For More Information: The Neponset District of the Metropolitan District Commission, 475 Neponset Avenue, Dorcester, Massachusetts 02122. Tel.: (617) 727-6034.

3. The Mystic River Reservation Bike Path

SOMERVILLE, MEDFORD, AND EVERETT, MASSACHUSETTS

General Description:

A 3.5-mile loop around the Mystic River, crossing the Wellington Bridge in Somerville.

Level of Difficulty: Easy.
Type of Scenery: The banks of the Mystic River; lots of traffic; very urban.
Condition of Pavement: Good

General Background:

This is one of the many paths maintained by the Metropolitan District Commission. It is almost impossible to find, unless you know exactly what you're looking for and precisely where to look for it. We asked for information at a state-police barracks on the Mystic River Reservation. None of the 3 officers we asked had heard there was a bike path on the Mystic River Reservation.

The Bike Path:

The path, it turned out, is quite lovely. In better shape than many MDC paths, the pavement snakes alluringly in and out of tall sedges bordering the wet banks of the Mystic River. At times, you're close enough to the riverbanks and far enough from the nearby parkway's automobile mayhem to enjoy a peaceful ride. Unfortunately, much of the pavement runs right alongside the heavy traffic, with no barrier separating cyclists from cars and trucks.

To ride this path for the first time, you ought to be in an exploratory mood. As on many of Boston's bike paths, the path appears to split at several points, but there are no signs to help you find your way. It's anybody's guess which is the main path and which leads to a dead end.

If you're looking for a bike path that doesn't get much use, consider this one. We visited the Mystic River Reservation Bike Path on the same Sunday afternoon that we visited the Minuteman Bikeway, barely a few miles distant. (See separate entry.) The much-touted Minuteman, with its myriad of signs and parking areas, had hundreds of visitors that day. On the Mystic River path, every bit as attractive (in places), we saw nary a cyclist. If you're looking for a bike path around Boston where you can work up some speed, a few spins around the Mystic River might fill the bill. (Don't ride alone here, however.)

Food Facilities Nearby: Plenty of nearby delis and fast-food places.

Restrooms: None.

Special Precautions: There's a reason why there's a state-police barracks on the Mystic River Reservation. Don't go there after dark. Boston's mystery writers like to mention the Mystic River as the place where murderers dump their bodies.

Best Parking Lot: The Mystic River Valley Parkway winds through the reservation. Along the way are well-marked parking areas. The bike path, not well marked, is nearby. You can often see it from the parkway.

Directions: Take Exit 30 off Interstate 93, and head east. You will be on Route 16, also called the Mystic Valley Parkway. Look for the bike path along the side of the parkway. When Route 16 changes names from the Mystic Valley to the Revere Beach Parkway, you've gone too far.

For More Information: The Mystic District of the Metropolitan District Commission, 1 Woodland Road, Stoneham, Massachusetts 02180. Tel.: (617) 662-8370.

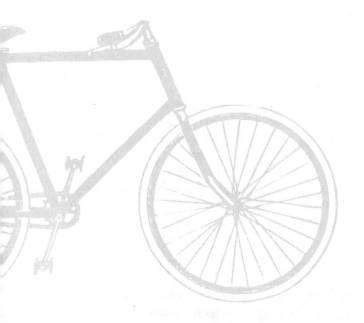

4. The Pierre Lallement Bike Path

SOUTHWEST CORRIDOR LINEAR PARK
BOSTON, MASSACHUSETTS

General Description:

A 4.7-mile, flat path through a unique urban park.

Level of Difficulty: Very easy.
Type of Scenery: Urban city scape; many road crossings.
Condition of Pavement: Excellent.

General Background:

Over the years, this transportation corridor has had many different intended purposes. In the early part of the nineteenth century, it was the Boston–to–New York railroad right-of-way. When the railroads declined, the corridor was slated to become a 12-lane highway, Interstate 95. About 100 acres of land had been cleared for that purpose by the early 1960s. Hundreds of buildings were razed and thousands of people moved to make way for the new highway, which would have sliced up the lower-income communities of Jamaica Plain, Roxbury, the South End, and the Back Bay.

In response, people lay down in front of the bulldozers. As the anti-interstate movement gathered steam, the people of those communities found numerous other ways to voice their disapproval. The 12-lane highway, they told city officials, would destroy the sense of community. In 1969, the government gave in. The state's governor, Francis Sargent, declared a moratorium on highway construction inside the Boston beltway, Route 128.

In the 1970s, a new plan was devised. The Orange Line of the "T," Boston's subway system, hanging in the air over nearby Washington Street like a menacing specter, was moved several blocks over, to this park, and built underground, allowing local residents easy access to the center of Boston. On top of that underground transportation system appeared a greenway—a corridor park with recreation areas, playgrounds, tennis courts, basketball courts. A walking path and a separate biking path appeared where the 12-lane highway was supposed to have gone.

The railway has become a 5-mile-long recreation corridor, a focal point for community spirit. The corridor begins in Boston proper, outside the very upscale Copley Place shopping mall. It ends in three different places: the Arnold Arboretum, with its collection of rare trees and plantings; at Franklin Park, with the nearby zoo; and at the Forest Hills subway stop.

Now a decade old, the park remains a source of community pride. More than 50,000 people visit daily, including about 1,000 bike commuters. The corridor looks as if it opened yesterday, thanks to the efforts of the more than 200 volunteers who provide maintenance services. Lawns are mowed. Trees are pruned and shrubs are sheered. Graffiti are removed. This volunteer group provides more than $125,000 a year in free services to the Southwest Corridor Park.

Boston's police headquarters sit on park premises. The 60-acre park also has community gardens, 2 street-hockey rinks, 5 tennis courts, spray pools, Little League playing fields, and 15 playgrounds for young children. The park is a model for city officials across the country who are trying to revitalize older urban areas.

The Bike Path:

The park's bike path was named after Pierre Lallement, who acquired the patent for the first pedal bicycle in the United States in 1866. Lallement sold his patent to the Pope Manufacturing Company of Boston in 1869. Pope manufactured the "Ordinary" bicycle—the bicycle with the huge front wheel and the awkwardly high seat—from 1871 to 1892.

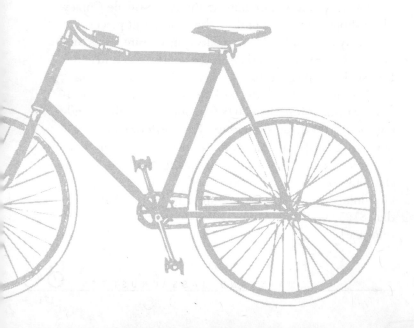

The Lallement is an urban bike path with many busy street crossings and lots of traffic noise. For people who live along its route, this is an excellent way to get in and out of the city. For visitors to Boston, however, it's not a particularly scenic way to enjoy the city. Most of the cyclists who use the path are commuters, but we suspect that anyone interested in the Greenway Movement might find it worth looking at.

Food Facilities Nearby: Lots of little sandwich shops and ethnic restaurants along the way.

Restrooms: None.

Special Precautions: Ride with a friend on this urban path after dark.

Best Parking Lot: This path can be accessed anywhere along the route, but parking will be difficult. A safe place to park is the mall parking lot at Copley Place in downtown Boston, although parking will be expensive.

Directions: To get to the beginning of the park at Copley Place, take the last exit off the Massachusetts Turnpike before Interstate 93. Follow signs to Copley Place.

For More Information: Southwest Corridor Linear Park, 38 New Heath Street, Jamaica Plain, Massachusetts 02130. Tel.: (617) 727-0057.

5. The Minuteman Bikeway

ARLINGTON, LEXINGTON, AND BEDFORD, MASSACHUSETTS

General Description:

A 10.5-mile rail trail that passes through several historic Massachusetts towns and ends in Bedford, the town that provided the Minuteman flag on April 19, 1775.

Level of Difficulty: Very easy.
Type of Scenery: Very urban in Cambridge; suburban in Arlington; almost rural in Lexington and Bedford.
Condition of Pavement: Excellent.

General Background:

This is a ride through the hotbed of the American Revolution! From Arlington to Lexington to Bedford, paralleling the road galloped at midnight by Paul Revere, the Minuteman cyclist rides through history. But unlike Revere, modern Minuteman riders can take the time out for a sunny picnic, visit a centuries-old house, read a historic marker, or just rest in a town green and watch the world go by.

The Minuteman Bikeway, named the 500th Rail Trail by the Rails-to-Trails Conservancy, was opened in 1992 after more than a decade of preparation. The bikeway, meant to encourage bike commuting in lieu of automobile commuting, runs from the Alewife subway station, the outermost station on the Red Line of Boston's subway system, to Bedford, an upscale and semi-rural town 10 miles to the northwest.

The railroad right-of-way first saw train travel in 1846, when the Lexington and West Cambridge railroad began train service from North Cambridge to Lexington. Twenty-five years later, when the railroad had become the Boston & Lowell Railroad, service extended all the way into Bedford. A century later, the railroad (now called the Boston & Maine) discontinued service.

Then came talk of extending the city's subway system along the railroad bed; these discussions were not met with enthusiasm on the part of nearby property owners. Instead, worried property owners suggested an alternative: a commuter-and-recreation bike path. As the years passed, this idea gained momentum.

The Minuteman is an immensely popular weekend recreation path. When we rode the path, one warm Sunday afternoon in December, it was as crowded as Route 128, the highway that circumnavigates the Bostonian metropolis. Unfortunately, a few of the path's weekend users behave quite like Route 128's manic drivers, who speed along the breakdown lane at 70 miles per hour, against all odds. We wish this weren't so.

Still, of all Boston's bike paths, the Minuteman is our favorite. It is the only path inside the Route 128 beltway that is well maintained, well marked, and well publicized. It is very easy to find, and is well separated from highways and roads for most of its length. Consequently, it is immensely crowded. If you want to ride fast, arrive early.

The Bike Path:

The path begins near the Alewife Brook Parkway, a.k.a. Route 16. There are several recreational fields near the intersection of Routes 16 and 2. If you want to begin biking here, either park at the Alewife subway stop, which will cost several dollars, or park near some of these recreational fields. Varnum Street and Lake Street, just off Massachusetts Avenue, are good parking possibilities.

We suggest, however, that you skip over this first section of the bikeway and park instead at Spy Pond, where you'll find a fairly large public parking area. Spy Pond, on the border of Cambridge and Arlington, was used in earlier centuries for ice harvesting. Throughout the long New England winters, workers cut huge chunks of ice and hauled them with teams of horses to nearby ice houses. From there the ice was shipped by railroad car, along the very railroad bed you'll be biking, to the Charlestown shipyards. Spy Pond ice traveled around the world, slated to melt in faraway lands like India and South America.

Today, Spy Pond is a pleasant urban-recreation area. During the warm months, sailing and wind surfing are allowed, although swimming is not. At the pond are a playground for younger children, picnic tables, and several acres of grassy parkland. The bikeway is easily accessible.

If you begin biking at Spy Pond, you'll soon come to the short section which requires walking along city sidewalks. In Arlington Center, bikeway officials ask you to walk your bike for several blocks through this congested area. (They really *do* want you, in the spirit of public cooperation, to do this; the bikeway is not separated from the public sidewalks, and shoppers get quite annoyed when they are run over by bikes or skaters.)

Bikeway planners were faced with the problem of pointing the way to the path in this congested area. We loved their solution: immense, colorful cloth banners with the Minuteman logo mark where the path picks up on both sides of Arlington Square. The huge flags, about 10 feet long and placed about 12 feet in the air above the path, give the whole area a rather festive look. You feel you're in some sort of Sunday-afternoon parade. By the way, if you're interested in historic houses, stop in Arlington Center and tour the Jefferson Cutter House, listed in the national historic register. Moved from its original location, the house is interesting to walk through.

Between Arlington and Lexington Center, a bit past the halfway point, you'll pass through several little park areas with picnic tables, swing sets, and rest areas set up for cyclists. Just before Lexington Center is the Arlington Reservoir, offering a mile-long walking path and a public swimming beach. This is a great place to stop, walk, and swim during the summer months.

Past the Arlington Reservoir, the bikeway becomes more rural. You'll cycle past the Cataldo Reservation and through Great Meadows, a wetland flowing into the reservoir. There are several points here where you can walk along side paths.

If you're biking the Minuteman for its historic interest, of course stop in Lexington Center. The nearby Lexington Visitor Center is open every day and will help you find the various historic sights in the town. You'll know you're in Lexington Center because the bikeway, just like the trains of old, passes underneath the overhang of an 1873 train shed.

On the other side of Lexington Center, the path passes the Route 128 beltway on a bridge built just for bikes. The bike path is now quite rural, which you'll notice by the flocks of foraging chickens blocking your way. There are plenty of cows on either side, too, as well as horse barns. The paved path ends on South Street, just before Bedford Center. Two unpaved railroad beds, one leading to Concord and the other to Billerica, extend from the end of the paved path. These are navigable on mountain bikes.

In-line skaters are welcome.

Food Facilities Nearby: In Arlington, Lexington, and Bedford centers, there are plenty of delis and inexpensive restaurants.

Restrooms: None.

Special Precautions: This much-publicized, well-designed path is so popular that Sunday afternoon traffic jams can resemble those on Route 128. Unfortunately, a few speedsters navigate along the Minuteman the way Boston drivers navigate Route 128.

Best Parking Lot: The bike path parallels Massachusetts Avenue almost from its beginning, at the Alewife subway stop in Cambridge, all the way to Lexington Center. If you drive this section of Massachusetts Avenue, you can see the path at many points. There are many parking possibilities along the way.

Spy Pond in Arlington is a particularly good place to park, with its large parking lot, picnic areas, and playground.

There is also a public parking lot in Lexington Center, beside the bike path. If you're making the Minuteman Bikeway part of a day's tour of Concord and Lexington, this is a good place to park and pedal.

Directions: To get to the Spy Pond parking lot, take Exit 29 (Route 2) from the Boston beltway, Route 128/I-95. Head east on Route 2. Turn left (east) on Route 16, also called the Alewife Brook Parkway. Turn left onto Massachusetts Avenue, heading toward Arlington Center. A small road on your left—Pond Lane—will lead to the park and the parking area.

To get to the Lexington Center parking lot, take the Lexington-Bedford exit, Routes 4 and 225. From the exit, head toward Lexington along Bedford Street. In the center of town, you'll pass the path on your left. The public parking area is on your left, just after Meriam Street.

For More Information: Planning & Community Development Department, Arlington Town Hall, 730 Massachusetts Avenue, Arlington, Massachusetts 02174. Tel.: (617) 641-4891.

Town Manager's Office, Lexington Town Offices, 1625 Massachusetts Avenue, Lexington, Massachusetts 02173. Tel.: (617) 861-2775.

Town Administrator, Bedford Town Hall, 10 Mudge Way, Bedford, Massachusetts 01730. Tel.: (617) 275-1111.

The Lexington Visitor Center, 1875 Massachusetts Avenue, Lexington, Massachusetts 02173. Tel.: (617) 862-1450.

6. The Jamaicaway Bike Path

General Description:

A 1.5-mile bike path that parallels the Jamaicaway automobile road, with another half-mile loop around a small freshwater pond.

Level of Difficulty: Average.

Type of Scenery: The 1891 parkland designed by Frederick Law Olmsted; Boston mounted police; a pretty little pond with a tiny island for ducks and geese; a busy, high-speed roadway.

Condition of Pavement: Excellent along the 1.5-mile stretch; half the loop around the pond is paved and the other half is well-packed cinder and gravel.

General Background:

A century ago, master landscape architect Frederick Law Olmsted, designer of New York's Central Park, envisioned a string of parklands running through Boston. Since each little park was like a tiny and delicate jewel, Olmsted's creation came to be called "The Emerald Necklace." Winding through these parks, to link his jewels, Olmsted designed bridle paths.

Around Jamaica Pond and along the Jamaicaway automobile road, Olmsted's wide and luxurious bridle paths are now paved, as horses have yielded to walkers and cyclists.

The parks themselves remain much the way Olmsted created them, with solid old stone buildings, with benches and huge trees, with playing fields and grassy lawns.

A century after their creation, Olmsted's parks are still wild refuges for beleaguered city residents. In fact, so many people walk around Jamaica Pond, even during the coldest winter months, that cyclists are asked *not* to ride around the pond itself, which is sad, because the path is beautiful and tempting.

The Bike Path:

Cyclists are welcomed, however, along a bike path that begins at the automobile rotary just south of Jamaica Pond. Like most Boston bike paths, this one is hard to find. It is marked with a small sign at its beginning, but the sign is too easy to miss. To find the bike path (as opposed to the *walking* path around the pond), stand at the rotary south of the pond and face the pond. The bike path will be on your right.

As you bike along this old bridle trail, you'll get a good idea of why people call Olmsted's design "a necklace." The bike path leads you from one sculpted park to another, until you arrive at tiny Leverett Pond, just south of Route 9. As you pedal around the quiet pathway that circles the pond, it's easy to forget about the busy road nearby. In the pond are tiny islands, some only a few feet in diameter. Waterfowl make their home in clumped sedges. Around the pond, majestic old hardwoods shield the park from the city's stresses and screen out the bright sun on a hot summer day.

There is more of Olmsted's necklace across Route 9,

but the peaceful cycling is interrupted here. Recreational cyclists will probably want to circle Leverett Pond and head back down the Jamaicaway cycling path. This ride— up the path, around Leverett Pond, back along the Jamaicaway path—is about 3.5 miles, round-trip distance.

Food Facilities Nearby: None near the bike path.

Restrooms: None.

Special Precautions: Part of this path parallels a busy road. Drivers completely ignore the speed limit, posted at 25; the *de facto* speed limit seems to be about 50. Since you're on a bike path, you won't be endangered, but you may find the noise and fumes annoying.

Best Parking Lot: Parking is allowed along the sides of the rotary just south of Jamaica Pond.

Directions: From Route 128, take Route 9 East to the Jamaicaway/Riverway parkway. Head southwest on the Jamaicaway, past Jamaica Pond, to the rotary. Enter the rotary to the right and park along the side near the pond.

For More Information: No contact address or telephone number.

7. Wompatuck State Park

General Description:

More than 3.5 miles of hilly paths and wide roads, built for trucks but now closed to motorized vehicles.

Level of Difficulty: Average to very challenging.

Type of Scenery: Stands of white pine and hemlock; small ponds and brooks; World War II bunkers and munitions facilities.

Condition of Pavement: Lots of cracking.

General Background:

During the nineteenth century, high-quality granite was quarried in this area, just south of Boston. Some large granite outcroppings exist in the park; in fact, cyclists on mountain bikes love to ride over these rock mounds. Because of the granite, there are also sudden and steep inclines. Prospect Hill rises from 120 to 240 feet above sea level in just over a quarter-mile. Consequently, Wompatuck State Park is a mecca for mountain bikers who want to get a good day's workout without traveling far from Boston. (The park is about a 15-minute drive from Route 128.)

During World War II, when Americans worried over U-boats, the military stored munitions here and built roads. Most of these roads are now closed to public motorized traffic. The wide roads and graded inclines make Wompatuck a great place for family cycling, since there's plenty of room to ride side by side.

The Bike Path:

The special paved bike paths and the wide roadways open to both walkers and cyclists make up an interconnected and often confusing network. Expect to get lost; you'll find your way eventually.

At many points, paved roads diverge in several different directions, as do cinder-covered side trails and dirt paths. Park officials have marked the paved bike paths with white arrows on the pavement and with blue arrows on the trees, but knowing which way to turn is often dicey, despite their efforts. Take a state trail map along with you. Available free at the Visitor Center, this has contour lines to help orient you, even if its bike-path and roadway lines don't.

There is also an intricate network of single-track dirt paths open to mountain cyclists.

Food Facilities Nearby: None.

Restrooms: Visitor Center.

Special Precautions: This forest respite in the midst of urban sprawl gets heavy use.

There are several very steep hills with unexpected sharp turns at the bottom.

Best Parking Lot: Visitor Center at the park's main entrance.

Directions: From Route 3, take Exit 14. Turn north on Route 228 and go through a set of traffic lights. State-park signs, brown with white lettering, will point the way. Travel along Route 228 for several miles, into the town of Hingham. Turn right on Free Street and go .8 mile. Turn right onto Union Street. A large state-park sign marks the turn. Pass through the entrance gate and up the hill to the large Visitor Center.

For More Information: Wompatuck State Park, Union Street, Hingham, Massachusetts 02043. Tel.: (617) 749-7160.

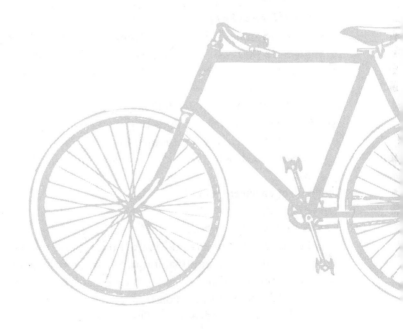

8. Myles Standish State Forest

CARVER AND PLYMOUTH, MASSACHUSETTS

General Description:

About 15 miles of tricky, intriguing trails running through a 15,000-acre state forest, one of the nation's largest pine-barren ecosystems. One of our favorite rides!

Level of Difficulty: Average to challenging.

Type of Scenery: Extensive stands of tall pines; many pond ecosystems; lots of wildlife, including the endangered Plymouth red-bellied turtle; coyotes, deer, osprey, and owls.

Condition of Pavement: Good.

General Background:

Massachusetts Forests and Parks builds some terrific bike paths. They twist and turn, requiring some proficient handling of bikes at times. The trails climb and drop with the precipitousness of roller-coasters, giving kids a special sense of back-country adventure. These meandering paths make full use of the region's rolling hills and are perfect for older kids who like challenge but aren't quite ready for on-road biking.

We love these paths—and the whole recreation area. It's a terrific place to spend a day, a weekend, or a week.

There's something for everyone: trails for hiking and biking, 35 kettle ponds for canoeing (no motorboats allowed), several sandy swimming beaches, almost 500 camping sites, and naturalist programs all summer long.

These forest expanses were once part of the Indian village of Patuxet. The Wampanoag granted them to the English settlers in 1621. Over the next 300 years, the forests were used in many ways, but failed to yield much profit. Though iron and peat were mined from the bogs, the resources weren't extensive. Forestry was tried, but the pine and scrub oak were not of good quality. Farming was impossible because the soil was too acidic.

Eventually, the land was designated wasteland. Beginning in 1916, the state began buying bits and pieces for recreational purposes, eventually assembling today's huge recreational area. During the Depression, the Civilian Conservation Corps built amenities like cabins and comfort stations.

The CCC also planted row after row of white pines, which have by now come of age. These forests are magical, mysterious, and enchantingly beautiful. Entering the stands of trees is like entering a cathedral. The shafts of light penetrate the forest as though filtered by stained-glass windows. On the forest floor is a carpet of fern-like green. Thousands of seedlings only a few feet high, nestled among the trunks of the mature trees, shimmer in the filtered light.

This is our favorite part of the forest, and, for some reason, few people use the paved path that penetrates this area. One summer Saturday, we biked its 4-mile length and met only a lone in-line skater, intrepidly climbing and coasting along over the steep, short hills.

The Bike Path:

Three separate paths run deep into the pine forests and curve around isolated ponds filled with plant and animal life. All 3 begin near park headquarters, branching out like spokes in a wheel to the northwest, northeast, and southwest.

Our favorite, described above, is the northwest path, probably a little more challenging than the other 2. Young cyclists not yet proficient with brakes and steering might not do well here. On the other hand, you'll encounter fewer people.

The trail that heads northeast from headquarters extends a bit more than 5 miles and is the most popular. There are some beautiful stands of trees along this path, but you won't see as much water. You must cross the most crowded of the automobile roads in the park several times. This trail ends at the opposite side of the park, at the eastern entrance.

The third trail is actually a group of trails of more than 5 miles that lace through the southwestern section of the park, looping around ponds and doubling back in confusing but interesting disarray. Lots of people like these trails: they climb and drop and include several water views. Lots of people also get lost on them. The park is not known for its efficient signage. Look for a stenciled "To Headquarters" sign painted in very faded white on the bike-path pavement. Don't start this ride too late in the day; it may take you some time to find your way back to headquarters.

Food Facilities Nearby: None, but there are ample picnic tables and scenic views.

Restrooms: Park headquarters.

Special Precautions: (1) These trails are closed during hunting season. Call ahead to be sure.

(2) The bicycle paths cross horse trails, dirt-bike trails, and automobile roads. Be sure children are aware of this. There are lots of horses in these forests. Some horses are terrified of bicycles and may rear or kick. Bikes always yield to horses.

(3) Watch out for high-speed cyclists zooming down the steep hills. The narrow paths and sharp turns make it difficult to see them. Stay on your own side of the path.

Best Parking Lot: At state-forest headquarters, intersection of Fearing Pond Road, Cranberry Road, and Lower College Pond Road.

Directions: (1) From Interstate 495, take Exit 2. Take Route 58 north for about 3 miles. Route 58 will veer sharply to the left; go straight. In about 1 mile, turn right onto Cranberry Road, which leads to the state-forest-headquarters parking lot, on the left. There will be brown state-park signs all along the route.

(2) From Route 3, take Exit 3; following signs for the state forest, head west, toward Long Pond Road; go right on Long Pond Road and head north until you see signs in the park to the headquarters parking lot, about 5 miles.

For More Information: Myles Standish State Forest, Cranberry Road, South Carver, Massachusetts 02366. Tel.: (508) 866-2526

9. Webb Memorial State Park

General Description:

About 1.25 miles of looped paths at the end of a neck of land extending into the Boston metropolitan-harbor area.

Level of Difficulty: Easy.

Type of Scenery: Great view of the downtown Boston skyline; oceangoing ship traffic; urban coastal views.

Condition of Pavement: Soft stone dust; sometimes difficult for narrow-tired bikes.

The Bike Path:

This 37-acre park is a scenic respite in the midst of the incredibly chaotic urban sprawl that lies directly south of Boston. The biking is limited, but at the outermost reach of the path are some great photography opportunities: Boston's harbor islands, sailboats and ships, the Boston skyline, and the lengthy urban coastline.

This is a good place to bring children who are just learning to bike. When they get tired of biking, there's plenty more here to interest them. The winds from the ocean make for fine kite flying. There are plenty of beaches to explore. (This is not a swimming area.) Sailboats and ships fill the nearby water. At the tip of the neck, just across the water, lies the city of Boston, with its distinctive downtown city skyline. It's a great place to get a perspective on the city as a whole.

Food Facilities Nearby: None.

Restrooms: None

Special Precautions: Can be windy. Sometimes becomes crowded.

Best Parking Lot: At the park entrance.

Directions: Near the Weymouth-Hingham line on Route 3A, look for the Weymouth Vietnam Memorial Park, a small park square on the ocean side of Route 3A. At the Vietnam park, turn onto Neck Street and drive a short distance down it to the Webb State Park parking lot.

For More Information: Boston Harbor Islands State Park, 349 Lincoln Street, Building 45, Hingham, Massachusetts 02043. Tel.: (617) 740-1605.

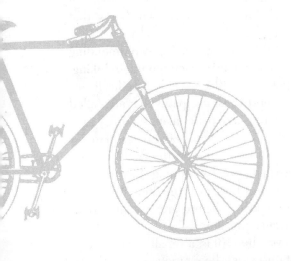

10. Bradley Palmer State Park

General Description:

A network of interlaced trails thread through this 721-acre state park.

Level of Difficulty: Very challenging.
Type of Scenery: Woodlands.
Condition of Pavement: A few cinder-and-gravel-covered trails; the remainder are dirt.

General Background:

Massachusetts distributes brochures which say that this state park has biking facilities.

We would hesitate, however, before recommending these trails for biking of any kind—even mountain biking. There are no paved paths, or paths set aside specifically for cycling. Instead, the cyclist must use paths that are called "hiking/bridle trails" on the state park's map.

During an hour's visit, we saw 30 horses. Horses inconvenience cyclists by chopping up the trails; cyclists inconvenience equestrians by frightening the animals. Considering the number of horses in the area, it seemed the hassle just wasn't worth it. There are so many other places to bike without such problems.

If you decide to cycle here (it is, after all, advertised as open to biking on state maps), be cautious of the horses and conscious of safety. The safest way to cope with horses is to stop your bike and stand until the animals pass.

This state park is connected to several large state forests, where you'll also encounter horses. An obvious solution would be for the state to build designated bike paths, separating bike riders from horseback riders.

Food Facilities Nearby: None.

Restrooms: None.

Special Precautions: Horses!

Best Parking Lot: At park headquarters.

Directions: Take Route 1 to Topsfield, turn onto Ipswich Road and travel 1.2 miles. Follow the brown state-park signs directing you to the park, only a few hundred yards away.

For More Information: Bradley Palmer State Park, Asbury Street, Topsfield, Massachusetts 01983. Tel.: (508) 887-5931.

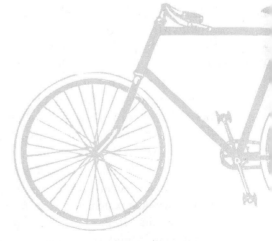

11. Lowell Heritage State Park

General Description:

A mile-long paved path along a particularly scenic section of the Merrimack River.

Level of Difficulty: Very easy.
Type of Scenery: A river ride through a very urban area.
Condition of Pavement: Excellent.

General Background:

With both a state and national historic park organized around the city's nineteenth-century textile mills, Lowell definitely merits a day's visit. But we were surprised to see on a state brochure that one of the activities offered is *cycling*.

When we arrived at the state-and-national-park area, we were even more surprised. None of the guides at either park had heard of a bike path. The parks offer trolley tours, walking tours, canal-barge tours—but we couldn't find biking anywhere. Finally, we found a National Park Service official who sent us out of the downtown area, across the Merrimack River, and then upstream to the Vandenberg Esplanade, a small bit of state parkland sandwiched in between busy Route 113 and the river.

Once we found it, we were surprised again. This tiny bit of riverside park is quite attractive. A dam just below the esplanade makes the river fine for sailing. A wide, paved recreation path, somewhat separated from the highway, runs along the water for just about a mile.

There's not really enough path to make the biking alone a destination, but if you're visiting the city's historic areas, a riverside lunch break and a short bike ride are a good way to get rid of museum fatigue.

Interestingly, there are several other places along the bank of the Merrimack River where recreation paths were once built. Unfortunately, to get to them from the state-park path, cyclists have to ride along the automobile highway. These riverside recreation paths are not marked with signs. Nor are they well maintained or connected to each other. We have heard some talk of upgrading the fragmented system, and of creating a much longer bike path along the river, but we have yet to find any concrete plans that look as if they might reach fruition.

Food Facilities Nearby: None.
Restrooms: At the esplanade during the summer months.
Special Precautions: Ride with a friend here.
Best Parking Lot: The Sampas Pavilion, Route 113.
Directions: From Route 3, Interstate 495, and Interstate 93, take the Lowell Connector all the way to the end. You will feed onto Central Street, in the middle of the city. Take Central Street left, toward the river, then turn right onto Bridge Street. Immediately on the other side of the river, turn left onto Route 113 (the VFW Highway). Travel upstream along the Merrimack River several miles. On your left, you will see brown state-park signs. Turn into the parking area

here. The trip from downtown to the esplanade requires only 5 to 10 minutes.

For More Information: No contact address or telephone number for this state park. Try the main Boston office: Massachusetts Department of Environmental Management, Division of State Parks and Forests, 100 Cambridge Street, 19th Floor, Boston, Massachusetts 02202. Tel.: (617) 727-3180 or (800) 831-0569.

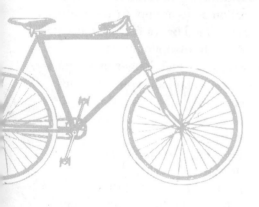

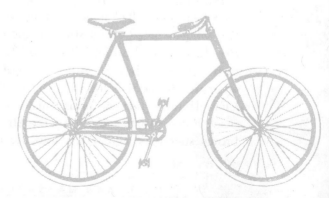

12. The Norwottuck Rail Trail

NORTHAMPTON, HADLEY, AND AMHERST, MASSACHUSETTS

General Description:

A mostly rural 8.5-mile rail trail, flat with very mild inclines, winding through attractive western Massachusetts farmland.

Level of Difficulty: Very easy.

Type of Scenery: A half-mile railroad bridge across the Connecticut River; several miles of village scenery and homes; open farmlands, marshes, and forests with mountains in the distance.

Condition of Pavement: Excellent.

General Background:

This rail trail, using the western end of the Central Massachusetts railroad line, opened in 1993. It runs through the Five College region of western Massachusetts and is state-of-the-art in rail-trail creativity. The public restroom at the trail's beginning in Elwell State Park has an environmentally sound non-flush toilet. Signs along the path remind riders that the paving material for the trail includes crushed glass recycled from the Materials Recovery Facility in nearby Springfield. Pete's Drive-In, an outdoor hamburger restaurant, is cyclist-friendly, offering first aid, restrooms, water, a picnic area, a swing set and a children's playground, tools for emergency bike repairs, even inner tubes and tire patch kits at cost.

There are as many in-line skaters and in-line cross-country skiers-on-wheels on this trail as there are cyclists. Some people do walk the trail, but not many; there are plenty of more interesting hiking trails in this region. The trail is forbidden to horses. We've seen officers on bicycles patrolling the trail. An elder-services organization brings seniors to walk the trail each month, beginning at the half-mile bridge over the Connecticut River.

There are dreams to extend this trail several miles at both ends, but it's difficult to say when—or if—it will happen. Despite the good will of many of the Norwottuck users, getting the trail approved by the various towns was an arduous undertaking. Frightened that the trail would bring an increase in vandalism, one town allocated $20,000 to fight the trail's construction in court. The money was never spent, but pockets of opposition remain strong in the town.

More than 40,000 people used the trail during its first year, and several thousand people use the trail each sunny summer weekend. Officials anticipate increases as more people learn of the trail's existence. Expect crowds.

The Bike Path:

This trail was first called the "Five College Rail Trail," but was renamed "Norwottuck" for the people who lived in the region before the Europeans arrived in the seventeenth century.

It begins at Elwell State Park, on the west bank of the Connecticut River just north of busy Route 9. The path begins by crossing a half-mile railroad bridge, now covered with wooden planks. Below is the 60-acre Elwell Island, one of the largest islands in the 410-mile-long Connecticut River. Elwell Island, owned by the Northampton Conservation Commission, is undeveloped. A variety of bird life and rare plants live in the island brush.

To the south is the Holyoke mountain range, which runs, oddly enough, east to west, rather than north to south. The most obvious peak visible from the railroad bridge is Mount Holyoke.

On the other side of the bridge is the town of Hadley, with its long and narrow town common. After this short urban section, the bike path enters fertile farmland and the tobacco fields which have determined so much of this area's social history. The tobacco grown here was a high grade used to wrap cigars. The long barns north of the bike path were drying sheds. Many of the immigrants who came from the Caribbean to pick at harvest time eventually settled in western Massachusetts and Connecticut.

This tremendously fertile, open farmland, surrounded by rugged mountains to the south, the north, and the west, is the result of a 157-mile lake that once stretched from Rocky Hill, Connecticut, all the way across Massachusetts to Hanover, New Hampshire. The lake was formed 16,000 years ago by meltwater from the last glacier, and drained 13,000 years ago, leaving behind soil any farmer in the Midwest would covet.

About two-thirds of the way through Hadley, the path tunnels under the road, then resurfaces and crosses Maple Street, where the Hampshire Mall and the Mountain Farms Mall are located. The path does pass near these malls, but remains somewhat separated from the shopping-center chaos.

Shortly after that, the path crosses the Hadley-Amherst town line, passes the Amherst Golf Course on the right, and then enters conservation areas with many hiking trails. The conservators of these areas would prefer that bikes not use most of the dirt trails. If you've brought a bike lock, you can leave your bike at the entrance to the hiking trail. There are town trail maps available, in case you want to know more about these walking trails.

Currently, the paved bike path ends at a small parking lot on Station Road in Amherst. The path continues from here, but is unpaved. People with mountain bikes do sometimes continue on.

Food Facilities Nearby: None at the Station Road end of the path. From Elwell State Park, the center of Northampton, with a variety of delis and ethnic restaurants, is about a mile away. Pete's, an outdoor hamburger restaurant along the bike path about 3 miles east of Elwell State Park, welcomes cyclists.

Restrooms: Environmentally sound outhouse only, with no running water, at Elwell State Park. Pete's Drive-In, about 3 miles from the railroad bridge, has a port-o-potty.

Special Precautions: Most of the accidents on this trail occur when high-speed cyclists run into slower riders or do not stop for traffic at road crossings.

If you want to avoid crowds, you must come early. By 10 A.M. on a rainy late-fall Sunday, this path was crowded with joggers, walkers, cyclists, skaters, skiers, baby carriages, and a dog or two.

Best Parking Lot: The biggest drawback of this bike path is problematic parking. The designated lots at Elwell in Northampton and Station Road in Amherst hold only a few cars. Path users have created some unhappiness in these neighborhoods by parking their vehicles on lawns, sidewalks, driveways, and roadways.

There is a designated parking lot at the Mountain Farms Mall, at the path's halfway point. Unfortunately, since it is halfway along the path, most people don't want to park here. Again, if you don't want to deal with parking problems, come early. Or, better yet: ride your bike to the path, if possible.

Directions: To get to the Elwell State Park parking lot, coming from Amherst and Hadley, cross the Connecticut River on the Route 9 bridge and turn right immediately onto Damon Road. You will immediately see the parking lot on the right.

To get to the Station Road parking lot in Amherst, from Route 9 turn south on South East Street and drive about 2 miles. Turn left onto Station Road and drive .9 mile. The parking lot is on your left.

For More Information: The Massachusetts Department of Environmental Management, P.O. Box 484, Amherst, Massachusetts 01004. Tel.: (413) 545-5993.

13. The Chicopee Memorial State Park

CHICOPEE FALLS, MASSACHUSETTS

General Description:
A 2.5-mile loop through lush, forested parkland.

Level of Difficulty: Average.

Type of Scenery: Freshwater pond and running stream; forest lands with mature stands of ash and birch, maple and oak, as well as red and white pine and tall hemlock.

Condition of Pavement: Good; in a few places, severe cracking.

General Background:

At the entrance of Chicopee Memorial State Park stand 15 dogwood trees, planted for the Chicopee servicemen who died in Vietnam.

This 574-acre park is a glittering jewel. At its center is a lovely little freshwater pond with a sandy swimming beach. Nearby is a picnic area with well-maintained green lawns and a large stand of tall, mature pine. A hiking trail circles the pond; the bike path veers off in another direction.

The Bike Path:

As is usual in the Massachusetts park system, the bike path is difficult to find. There are some signs, but they are notably vague. To find the path, if you park in the lot closest to the pond, stand facing the pond. To your left, leading from the parking area and running along the pond, is a paved road wide enough to accommodate automobile traffic. This is closed to public traffic, although you will see park vehicles at times.

Begin biking here. The wide avenue travels along the pond past beachfront buildings, then past the dam and through stands of gracefully bowed white birch. A narrow paved trail leads up the hill to the left; this is not a bike path, but ends at a parking area above the path. Continue along the wide avenue. You'll coast down a hill and over a small bridge crossing the brook.

The loop begins by climbing steeply. Don't be dissuaded. This is the only truly difficult hill. At the top, the path levels out and circles around through peaceful forestland. At the other end of the loop, you descend a hill to return to the green bridge and the wide avenue that runs by the swimming pond to the parking lot.

Within the boundaries of this unusual park, the landscape is serene, almost rustic. Yet the park lies in the very urban Springfield-Chicopee region. On a Saturday afternoon in the fall, after the swimming season, this park was nearly empty, but during the summer, families from the nearby towns come to swim, picnic, and cycle. If you come on a summer day, arrive early and expect crowds. If you come on a fall or spring day just to bike, you may feel as though you own the place.

Food Facilities Nearby: None. Bring your own picnic.

Restrooms: At park headquarters, when open for swimming during the summer months.

Special Precautions: This park has specific daily opening and closing hours. The main gate, the only way to get in or out with an automobile, is locked during closing hours. Hours are seasonal; the park is usually open from 8 A.M. or 9 A.M. until dark, but if you want to come early or late in the day, or during the winter months, call first to be sure the park is open.

During the summer months, parking is $2 per car.

Best Parking Lot: During the summer months, the main parking lot, by the pond, fills up quickly. There are several large overflow parking lots, but on hot days these fill up also. If it's prime swimming weather, arrive early or expect to wait.

Directions: This park is less than 5 minutes by car from the Massachusetts Turnpike. Take Exit 6 off the pike. Turn right after the toll booths, onto Burnett Road. Travel less than a half-mile. The park is on your left, well marked. The address is 570 Burnett Road.

For More Information: Park headquarters tel.: (413) 594-9416.

14. Wendell State Forest

General Description:

At least 20 miles of rutted dirt roads through rugged forests, described in state brochures as "bike paths" but really ought to be called bike "trails," since they are more suitable for mountain biking.

Level of Difficulty: Very challenging. One dirt road designated a "bike path" drops more than 600 feet in less than a mile.

Type of Scenery: Almost 8,000 acres of undeveloped, mountainous forestlands.

Condition of Pavement: Rugged dirt roads with rocks and tree roots.

General Background:

A few of the dirt roads through this state forest have been officially designated "bike paths," but when we visited them we couldn't really tell why. These "paths" are really just wide roads, deeply rutted and not at all suitable for any but mountain bikes.

If you have a mountain bike, and you enjoy negotiating tree roots and boulders, this is a great place to visit. It is not a great place, however, for inexperienced back-country cyclists. The terrain is too rough and the mountains are too steep for most people. Without a well-designed mountain bike, you could easily bend a wheel.

If you want to try, definitely visit forest headquarters for advice. They will give you, among other things, a map of the state forest with contour lines—crucial when you're deciding where to ride. The map will also help you with the confusingly interlaced road system. It's incredibly easy to get lost in this expanse.

Food Facilities Nearby: None.

Restrooms: At state-forest headquarters, during the summer months.

Special Precautions: This is semi-wilderness state forest, far from hospitals, towns, restaurants. Bring your own first-aid supplies.

The state forest is officially "closed," meaning the main gate is locked, during some fall and spring months. While this means park headquarters is closed, cyclists may use the dirt roads that crisscross the forest at any time of the year. In the winter, this is a snow-mobile mecca.

Best Parking Lot: There are many places to park: on the sides of roads or at the beginning of dirt trails. Facilities and a parking lot are located at forest headquarters, along with the necessary contour maps.

Directions: From Route 2, take Route 63 South through Millers Falls. Take Wendell Road over the railroad bridge, turn onto Montague Road, and follow the signs for the state forest. The signs are sometimes difficult to notice at the intersections, but if you follow them faithfully, they will lead you to headquarters.

For More Information: State-forest headquarters tel.: (413) 659-3797. For trail map, send a self-addressed and stamped envelope to the Massachusetts Department of Environmental Management, Division of State Parks and Forests, Wendell State Forest, Wendell Road RFD #1, Millers Falls, Massachusetts 01349.

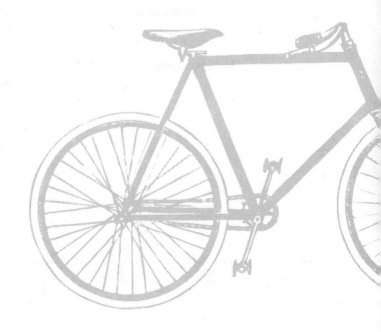

If you have information about a bike path

that ought to be included in this series, please contact:

Wendy Williams

P.O. Box 14

Mashpee, Massachusetts 02649

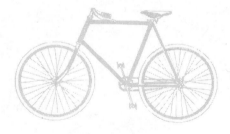